The HRT-Free Menopause Breakthrough

The HRT-Free Menopause Breakthrough

New Natural Alternatives

Marilyn Glenville, Ph.D.

Foreword by JoAnn V. Pinkerton, M.D.

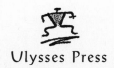

Ulysses Press

Published by Ulysses Press
        P.O. Box 3440
        Berkeley, CA 94703
        www.ulyssespress.com

First published as *The New Natural Alternatives to HRT* in Great Britain in 2002 by Kyle Cathie Limited

ISBN 1-56975-357-1
Library of Congress Control Number: 2003104410

U.S. editor: Richard Harris
U.S. editorial and production: Lily Chou, Claire Chun, James Meetze, Lynette Ubois

Printed in Canada by Transcontinental Printing

10 9 8 7 6 5 4 3 2 1

Distributed in the United States by Publishers Group West

Disclaimer

This book has been written and published strictly for informational purposes, and in no way should it be used as a substitute for consultation with your medical doctor or health care professional. All facts in this book came from medical files, clinical journals, scientific publications, personal interviews, published trade books, self-published materials by experts, magazine articles, and the personal-practice experiences of the authorities quoted or sources cited. You should not consider educational material herein to be the practice of medicine or to replace consultation with a physician or other medical practitioner. The author and publisher are providing you with information in this work so that you can have the knowledge and can choose, at your own risk, to act on that knowledge. The author and publisher also urge all readers to be aware of their health status and to consult health professionals before beginning any health program, including changes in dietary habits.

All names and identifying characteristics of real persons have been changed in the text to protect their confidentiality.

*To all women who want to
take responsibility for their health*

Author's Acknowledgements

This book was originally planned simply as a revised version of the first *Natural Alternatives to HRT*. But after looking at the huge amount of information that has emerged since its publication, I quickly realized that the writing was going to take much longer. I am therefore very grateful to my office staff, especially Linda McVan, my practice manager, for being so efficient and well organized, and thereby freeing up my time.

I would also like to thank Linda Gray for reading through the manuscript and asking questions where needed, and Catherine Blake, my editor. My special thanks go to Kyle, who way back in 1997 saw that women needed to know about the alternatives to HRT.

My warmest appreciation goes to Mr. Yehudi Gordon, consultant gynecologist, with whom I work very closely. He also believes that women should be given choices around menopause and that they should be offered the best of both conventional and nutritional medicine. By combining the best diagnostic tools of conventional medicine with the holistic approach of nutritional medicine, women can feel that they have the best of both worlds.

And of course my love and appreciation goes to my family, Kriss, Matt, Len and Chantell, for their constant support and encouragement.

Contents

Foreword

In 1997, the National Institutes of Health (NIH) sponsored a large randomized clinical trial of Hormone Replacement Therapy (HRT) for menopausal women. The study, pitting a combination of estrogen and progesterone against a placebo, was stopped in 2002, three years early, because of a finding of an increased risk of adverse health effects. This study led to panic among women on HRT and large numbers of women elected to go off their medications.

What we learned from this trial was that the type of HRT tested in this study did not prevent heart disease. In fact, the findings showed a small increase in heart events in the study's HRT users compared to those taking the placebo. We also found an increase in the risk of breast cancer, which was also found in the Million Women Study in Britain.

These studies have caused many of us to rethink why women are taking hormones and how long they should stay on them. For example, women who have been on HRT for five years or more, particularly if they are taking hormones primarily to prevent heart disease, should consider tapering off HRT. There are other ways to prevent heart disease, such as making lifestyle and diet changes.

Specific decisions about whether you need HRT or can rely completely on natural alternatives should, of course, be made with the help of your health care practitioner. Every women needs adequate amounts of calcium, vitamin D and other nutrients, a diet low in cholesterol and saturated fats, and regular aerobic exercise along with exercise against resistance, such as weight-training. It's also important to assess, along with your health care practitioner, your personal risk and fear of breast cancer, osteoporosis, and heart disease.

In this book, Dr. Marilyn Glenville provides a comprehensive summary of natural options for menopausal problems. She guides you through these questions and provides a wealth of information to help you to make the best decisions possible about your path through menopause. Remember, in the long run, your health is in large part up to you.

JoAnn V. Pinkerton, MD
Director of The Women's Place: Midlife Health Center
Associate Professor, Obstetrics and Gynecology
University of Virginia Health Sciences Center

Preface

In the U.S. a large proportion of women take Hormone Replacement Therapy and a number of prominent medical practitioners are enthusiasts of HRT. One gynecologist, for example, suggests that all women after menopause should take supplementary hormones.

This book is not meant to disparage doctors; there are many women who receive sound advice regarding menopause from their medical practitioners. In fact, many doctors are now aware of the importance of nutrition in a person's health, and have adopted a sympathetic approach to menopause and treat it as a natural stage in a woman's life. However, the women I see, almost without exception, have not been happy with the recommendations given to them.

It is my hope that those doctors who routinely recommend HRT, and consider menopause an illness, will be made aware of the facts contained in this book – facts that may not have been brought to their attention before. I hope that I have presented these facts in such a way that patients and doctors alike will consider that there are natural, safe and effective ways to care for women's health.

★

I originally published a book on HRT in Britain in 1997, *Natural Alternatives to HRT*, which quickly became an international bestseller. The book's reception revealed the enormous interest in the natural approach that exists worldwide. It proved that women desperately wanted to know what choices were available to them so they could make informed decisions about their health and lifestyle.

In the process of researching the *HRT-Free Menopause Breakthrough* I have uncovered some startling issues hidden in the medical literature, which I feel all women should be made aware of. Can phytoestrogen supplements (soy and red clover) increase the risk of breast cancer? Are new "designer" HRTs safe? Does HRT increase the risk of Deep Vein Thrombosis on flights? Do mammograms cause more deaths than they save? In my original book I put forward my opinion that HRT could increase a woman's risk of heart disease and breast cancer. This has since been borne out by the news that large-scale trials using HRT have been stopped because the risks were too great. It is now acknowledged that not only does HRT increase the risk of breast cancer, contrary to the previous advice, it does not prevent heart disease or strokes and may actually increase the risk.

I thought it was important to explain the controversy surrounding HRT and osteoporosis in this new book so that women can be fully aware of what the research actually shows (which may bear little resemblance to what they have been told).

Women today want to be well informed so that they can participate in making decisions about managing their symptoms, despite the fact that numerous papers have been written on how to make women more "compliant" – in other words, to encourage them to continue taking HRT.[1] Although there is pressure on women to go on HRT even before their periods have stopped, they are increasingly uneasy about taking it and there is a high dropout rate. Almost 40 percent stop using HRT within eight months, and 50 percent ask to change treatments at least twice. Modern women are far from "compliant." Their questions come hard and fast: "What is the benefit of taking this treatment?"; "What are the possible side effects and are there any risks?"; "What happens if I decide not to take this drug?" And most important of all, "What other choices do I have?"

This book is all about choices – knowing what is available and being able to use that information. Each woman is an individual with her own medical history and risk factors, so an important part of *HRT-Free Menopause Breakthrough* aims to help you determine whether you are at high risk of health problems such as osteoporosis and heart disease. This knowledge is important for any woman managing menopause or considering HRT. As with all medication, you must measure the risks against the benefits. If you discover that you can control menopausal symptoms naturally, why would you want to take HRT? Surely it is better to work at keeping yourself healthy to prevent problems in the future, monitoring your health regularly so you can review your decision if things change.

Too many doctors see women as a collection of hormones and thus regard menopause as a deficiency disease that needs to be corrected by replenishing declining levels of estrogen. Always bear in mind, however, that it is not an illness requiring treatment but a natural event in a woman's life. Given the right tools, diet, nutrition, and lifestyle, your body can adapt to this change naturally, efficiently, and comfortably, without the risks and side effects of HRT.

Author's Note

Hormone Replacement Therapy, in varying forms, has been around since the 1930s but over the last decade it was seen as the panacea for everything. The menopausal woman has been led to believe that HRT would not only help with hot flashes and night sweats, but also improve her memory, her sleep, and her sex life while giving her more energy and making her feel happier. More importantly, many women feared that without HRT, they were at risk for heart disease.

However, during the first years of the 21st century an explosion of research has been released negating the health benefits of HRT.

The new reality of HRT is that it has more risks than benefits because it can increase the risk of heart disease and breast cancer. Research now suggests that it does not do the very things that women took it for in the first place. HRT does not improve quality of life by improving memory, energy, sex drive or depression and it has now been found to increase the risk of Alzheimer's disease and other forms of dementia.

With this new information, it is even now more important for women to know that there are natural alternatives to HRT that eliminate the common symptoms of menopause such as hot flashes and night sweats. And that by using these natural remedies you can help improve the quality of your life while at the same time not risk a serious illness like breast cancer or heart disease.

Menopause is a natural event in a woman's life. It is not an illness. You need to know what choices are available to make informed, intelligent decisions that take you through this natural transition comfortably, without the need for powerful drugs and the side effects we now know these drugs carry. That is why this book was written.

CHAPTER 1

What Is Menopause?

Menopause happens because you have literally run out of eggs. Your store of eggs is already in place when you are born. Most women are born with about 2 million egg follicles; by puberty there are about 750,000, and by the age of around 45, only 10,000 may be left. The rest have disintegrated over the years. Menopause occurs when your store of eggs runs dry.

Strictly speaking, menopause is your very last period. What is generally referred to as menopause is actually the "climacteric," which is medical jargon for the transition period, which may span 15 to 20 years. A more helpful description might be the traditional one, the "change of life," since these years divide into three distinct phases:

1. Pre-menopause – periods are still regular but the first symptoms, such as hot flashes and mood changes, may appear.
2. Peri-menopause – the function of the ovaries declines, the periods can become irregular and symptoms may be more severe.
3. Post-menopause – your final period and beyond.

What's happening to your hormones?

One sign that menopause is approaching is a surge in follicle-stimulating hormone (FSH). This hormone causes the follicles in the ovaries to grow and is released every month in a normal cycle. In the run-up to menopause, the number of cycles in which eggs are not released increases. Estrogen begins to decline during the first two weeks of the cycle and ovulation becomes less likely, although you can still have periods. Without rising levels of estrogen to send a message back to the ovaries telling them to produce smaller amounts of FSH, the levels of FSH in the bloodstream keep growing as your body registers that ovulation is not taking place.

This increase in FSH levels can be measured by blood or urine tests (see page 213) to help to detect the onset of menopause. As you go through menopause, FSH levels become progressively higher and although levels can vary from month to month, the amount of FSH in your body is a relatively

The monthly cycle

During your fertile years, a number of reproductive hormones, such as estrogen, progesterone, follicle-stimulating hormone (FSH) and luteinizing hormone (LH), come into play at different times in the month.

The first day of your period is also the first day of your next menstrual cycle. On this day, FSH is released from the pituitary gland.

FSH stimulates the growth of a group of follicles on the surface of the ovary. These follicles will eventually produce eggs.

Over the next two weeks (the "follicular phase" of the cycle), the eggs grow and mature. At the same time, levels of estrogen, the leading female hormone, begin to rise.

As estrogen levels increase, the pituitary gland decreases its production of FSH. Another hormone, known as luteinizing hormone (LH) is triggered. Fertile alkaline mucus is produced in the cervix to keep sperm alive and to encourage their transportation through the cervix and up toward the Fallopian tubes, where fertilization can take place.

As LH surges, a mature egg (normally only one, but sometimes more) is released from a follicle and enters the Fallopian tube. This is known as ovulation.

The empty follicle (or "corpus luteum") begins to produce the second major female hormone, progesterone. The second half of the cycle (the "luteal phase") has begun.

If fertilization occurs, the fertilized egg will travel down the Fallopian tube and implant in the lining of the uterus (the endometrium). If fertilization does not take place, the lining of the uterus breaks down and is expelled. This is your normal monthly period. At the same time, there is a rapid and dramatic fall in the levels of estrogen and progesterone. With this drop in hormone levels, the cycle starts all over again.

good measure of the stage you have reached. You may also become aware that some of the signs you normally associate with ovulation are absent and you may start to experience symptoms of menopause such as hot flashes and night sweats, which can all start well before your periods stop.

Estrogen is still produced by the ovaries for at least 12 years after the start of menopause, although in much smaller quantities than before (so the menopausal ovary is certainly not a "dead" or "dying" organ, as popular opinion would still have it). The adrenal glands (which sit on top of the kidneys) also produce estrogen, which replenishes the ovaries' diminishing supply. Body fat is another manufacturing plant for estrogen, which is why it is not healthy to crash-diet and lose weight rapidly, especially during menopause. It is fine to become slightly heavier at this time because the extra estrogen from the fat cells helps to compensate for the declining amount produced by the ovaries. A fatter post-menopausal woman can produce more estrogen than a skinny pre-menopausal woman.

Nature is always trying to maintain a balance because estrogen levels that are too high or too low can play havoc with the body. While being too thin and producing too little estrogen can make the bones vulnerable to osteoporosis, being very overweight triggers excess estrogen levels, which increase the risk of breast and uterine cancer. This is because some types of breast and uterine cancer are estrogen-sensitive, meaning that estrogen can stimulate cancer cells and help them to grow. Estrogen is one of the body's builders, helping to form the lining of the uterus in the second half of the cycle and protecting the bones. However, if this building mechanism goes out of control, increased cell growth may lead to an estrogen-dependent cancer.

High levels of estrogen are also responsible for other painful, although not life-threatening, conditions. These include endometriosis (when the lining of the uterus grows in places other than just the uterus), fibroids (benign growths in the uterus), heavy and/or long periods and fibrocystic breast disease (lumpy and tender breasts).

Estrogen – the three-in-one hormone

Estrogen is not just one hormone, but three – estradiol, estrone and estriol – all of which have beneficial effects on the skin and vagina and protect the heart and bones.
• Estradiol, the most potent form of estrogen, 80 times stronger than estriol, the weakest type, is secreted by the ovaries. It is very active during adolescence but as menopause approaches, it declines.
• Estrone is produced by the adrenal glands and estrogen-manufacturing fat cells, which continue to release it after menopause. It is 12 times stronger than estriol.
• Estriol is the weakest form of estrogen and it is converted from estradiol (the most carcinogenic estrogen) and estrone (less carcinogenic) by the liver.

When do women reach menopause?

The average age in the U.S. is 51, which means that as many women go through menopause before this age as afterward. On the face of it, it would seem more beneficial to have a late menopause because the female hormones play an important part in protecting the bones. But a woman who is still menstruating around the age of 55 should have a checkup in case there is a medical reason for her continuing periods, such as fibroids (see "Late menopause," below).

The timing of menopause can be linked to a number of factors. The age at which your mother reached menopause can be a good guide. However, your experience of the symptoms may be quite different from hers, so even if she had a difficult time, there is no reason to fear that you will suffer in the same way. As you will see, there are plenty of things you can do to improve your health and control what is happening.

EARLY MENOPAUSE
• Smokers tend to have an earlier menopause, by about two years on average, because smoking diminishes the secretion of estrogen in the ovaries.
• A hysterectomy, even without the removal of the ovaries, can accelerate the onset of menopause by about five years. It is believed this happens because of the change in the supply of blood to the ovaries after surgery.
• Sterilization, where the Fallopian tubes are cut as a contraceptive measure, can bring on an earlier menopause for the same reason.

LATE MENOPAUSE
• Women who are overweight can have a later menopause because of the extra estrogen manufactured by the fat cells.
• Women who have fibroids (benign growths in the uterus) may experience a later menopause because they produce higher levels of estrogen. Although fibroids can be removed surgically, this is not always necessary because they frequently shrink at menopause when estrogen levels drop. Unfortunately women sometimes find themselves in a Catch-22 situation, where the estrogen excess that allows the fibroids to grow delays the drop in hormone levels needed to make them shrink.

HOW WILL YOUR PERIODS STOP?
The way your periods stop is as varied as the timing of menopause. They may stop abruptly; even though your cycle has been perfectly regular, one month your period doesn't appear and you never have another one. Sometimes

periods are regular but bleeding becomes shorter and shorter until it stops. Other women experience irregular bleeding and often periods become heavier but with gaps of several months in between.

SUDDEN MENOPAUSE

Menopause doesn't always go according to plan. Surgical intervention, an unusually small supply of eggs and even stress can all make it a sudden rather than a gradual change.

Surgical menopause

Surgical menopause occurs after the ovaries have been removed (a procedure called "oophorectomy"). This is obviously necessary if the ovaries are diseased, but often healthy ovaries are taken out as a routine measure during a hysterectomy.

If the ovaries are taken out before menopause has taken place, the effect can be traumatic for you and your body because it then arrives literally overnight. As soon as the ovaries are removed, the female hormone supply from the ovaries is cut off. And apart from plunging you into menopause, an oophorectomy can also cause a loss of libido, since during a natural menopause the ovaries continue producing testosterone, the hormone that helps with sex drive and arousal. HRT is usually prescribed to prevent the onset of menopausal symptoms.

Contrast this sudden withdrawal of estrogen with what happens during a natural menopause. Nature intends things to be taken gradually so that your body can adjust at its own pace and menopause can be a smooth change in your life. This can still happen after a hysterectomy if you retain your ovaries: menopause progresses naturally and can take anything from 15 to 20 years as hormone levels gradually decline.

Why, you might ask, are gynecologists so eager to remove healthy ovaries? Women who are about to have a hysterectomy are often advised to have them taken out "just in case" – in other words, removing them will prevent any possibility of ovarian cancer. Many doctors believe that as your uterus is being removed, you will no longer be able to have children so why hang onto your ovaries? Why not clear out the whole "works" at the same time, to "tidy you up"?

This may sound like a sensible approach but the thinking behind it is undoubtedly flawed. The American College of Obstetricians and Gynecologists has estimated that 700 ovaries would have to be removed to prevent a single case of ovarian cancer.[1] Yes, ovarian cancer is one of those "silent killers" and it is not easy to detect. Unless there is a strong family history of the disease, however, there is very little, if any, value in removing the ovaries during a hysterectomy.

You may be surprised to hear me suggesting that HRT might be useful, but it is important to remember that a surgical menopause is not a natural menopause. If you are under 40 and have had a surgical menopause, you could be at greater risk of osteoporosis, and HRT (which would be given as estrogen only) may be a sensible option. However, you should still adopt all the nutritional recommendations set out in the following chapters so that when you reach 50 or thereabouts, you could then talk to your doctor about coming off HRT, as this would have been the approximate age for your menopause anyway.

Some young women in this situation have come to my clinic needing to come off HRT because of the side-effects. It is important that they have both bone density and bone turnover monitored (see page 89) on a regular basis, to help prevent osteoporosis, and to keep as healthy as possible through diet, supplements and exercise.

If you are over 40 and have had a surgical menopause, the situation is different. My suggestion would be to have both bone density and bone turnover measured to find out where you stand. If your bone density is good, then use the recommendations in this book to control the menopausal symptoms and prevent osteoporosis. If you are showing signs of osteoporosis already, then you need to discuss with your doctor whether it would be more prudent to opt for medication that is specifically for the bones (see page 90) rather than HRT.

Premature menopause

This is a menopause that happens naturally before the age of 40. Also called premature ovarian failure, it is estimated to affect a minimum of 250,000 women in the U.S., some still in their teens and early 20s. In my practice, I have seen women as young as 17 who have experienced premature menopause. Periods start normally and then, after a couple of years, suddenly stop. Until recently, this problem did not receive much attention and, as a result, was often missed. Fortunately there is now much greater awareness and organizations such as the Daisy Network (daisynetwork.org.uk) and the Premature Ovarian Failure Support Group (www.pofsupport.org) have been set up to support women who are affected.

Premature menopause is usually diagnosed by a combination of blood tests and scans. As young women should have comparatively low levels of FSH, a high reading can be an indication of a premature menopause. A battery of tests can be performed to rule out other problems such as Polycystic Ovary Syndrome (which can be treated).

It can be devastating for a young woman whose periods have stopped to discover that she has reached menopause. Not only does it make having a baby impossible without the use of donor eggs, but it also means she has to cope with problems such as hot flashes, vaginal dryness and, even more dangerous for a young woman, osteoporosis.

Any woman in this position will need to discuss the use of hormone replacement therapy. Again, it may seem odd that I should consider HRT a useful option, but it is important to bear in mind that premature menopause is a medical condition because it is not happening at the usual time. It means that a young woman will be short of essential female hormones for up to 30 years longer than normal. These hormones are important for the bones as well as for preventing many of the other symptoms that can occur around menopause, such as vaginal dryness and hot flashes.

What causes premature menopause? It can be triggered by radiotherapy, and there is research to show that the condition is also related to smoking. Scientists have discovered that substances in cigarette smoke called polycyclic aromatic hydrocarbons can be toxic to a woman's eggs and make them die at a faster rate than normal, so pushing a woman faster into menopause. In 70 percent of cases, however, there is no medical explanation.

If there is no medical reason for your premature menopause and a scan indicates that your ovaries look healthy, it is well worth using the natural approach to try to get your periods back. (This subject is covered in great detail in my book *Nutritional Handbook for Women*.) From my experience, the sooner you do something about the problem, the greater the chance that the natural approach will work – in other words, if you start treatment as soon as possible

---

Reversing menopause naturally

Susan, a healthy 40-year-old woman, came to see me because her periods had suddenly stopped. She had been to see her doctor and blood tests showed she was menopausal. She was getting hot flashes and was concerned because she felt she was a "bit too young" to be going through menopause. I asked her what had been happening around the time that her periods ceased and she said that she had lost her job and had also lost her father.

I explained that the aim would be to ensure that she was as healthy as possible, addressing any problems with her diet, checking out any vitamin and mineral deficiencies, working on her stress levels and using herbs to help balance her hormones. She was happy with this approach

continued

because she believed that attaining optimum health would make her feel much better, regardless of whether her periods came back. Within a couple of months, her periods had returned and a further test at her doctor's showed that she was no longer "menopausal."

During times of stress, either physical (extreme weight loss, for example) or emotional (bereavement), the body starts to shut down the reproductive system in order to give you the resources you need to cope with what is going on. Because Susan was able to address the cause of her lack of periods, her body quickly kicked back into action.

Surprise pregnancy

You do need to be careful to avoid unwanted pregnancy in the years before menopause – and remember, HRT is not a contraceptive. Although ovulation is absent in an increasing number of cycles, it can occur intermittently, and periods can come and go erratically, so you could become pregnant and be completely unaware of it. Certainly fertility declines dramatically during your forties, but pregnancy is a very real possibility.

An interesting story in the *Journal of the British Menopause Society* (June 2001) describes a 49-year-old widow whose husband had been dead for ten months. Since his death her periods had become irregular and by the time she visited her doctor she had had no periods for six or seven months. She complained about abdominal swelling and pain under her lower ribs and her doctor thought she had gall bladder problems. However, a scan soon showed that she was 22 weeks pregnant. She was devastated. Apparently she had conceived after being "comforted" by an old friend.

As a rough guide:

If you are under 50, wait for two years after your periods have stopped before you give up contraception. If you are over 50, wait for one year.

after your periods stop and your condition is diagnosed, it is more likely that your periods will return.

*

Nature takes her time, she does things gradually. The change of life is a gradual process allowing your body to get used to the changes and to adapt accordingly. If your body is healthy, these changes can happen smoothly and comfortably.

CHAPTER 2

What Are the Symptoms of Menopause?

Not all women have a miserable time during menopause. Symptoms can vary and some women sail through – the only thing they notice is that their periods have stopped.

This in itself proves how illogical it is to see menopause as a deficiency disease caused by falling hormone levels. If it were some sort of disease, then all women would experience menopause in the same way, whereas in fact the symptoms can differ enormously from woman to woman, and can also be determined by cultural differences. Clearly, then, other factors are involved besides declining levels of hormones.

Too often modern gynecology homes in on the symptoms of menopause and tries to correct those instead of looking at the body as a whole. In fact, the change of life is a gradual process and the hormone systems in your body are interlinked and work in harmony with each other. Hormones introduced at menopause in the form of HRT are actually overriding what is happening naturally – these hormones should not be there at this time so HRT should not be called a "replacement" therapy. The condition of menopause is very different from a deficiency disease such as diabetes, when the pancreas does not produce insulin. Someone suffering from this illness needs insulin replaced because it isn't there when it should be.

At menopause, the body has to cope with the introduction of these external hormones in the form of HRT at a time when naturally it is reducing its own supply of them. Unfortunately, this is likely to have unwanted consequences. That is why women should think twice about taking HRT and ask what can be done to help them through this transition naturally, efficiently and comfortably, helping the body to balance itself.

None of this is to deny that there are many women who need help to cope with their symptoms. Some women who come to my clinic report being drenched in sweat 24 hours a day. They may have to get up to change their clothes two or three times a night, and some even find themselves taking a shower in the small hours.

Menopause or mid-life crisis?

First of all it is important to discover which symptoms, if any, are truly menopausal. All of the following are frequently blamed on menopause:

- hot flashes
- night sweats
- irritability
- declining libido
- osteoporosis
- weight gain
- vaginal dryness
- aging skin
- headaches
- mood swings
- depression
- lack of energy
- joint pains
- hair loss and changes in hair quality

The truth is that many of these so-called "menopausal symptoms" may have little to do with menopause. Some are just a natural part of the aging process and affect middle-aged men just as much as they affect women – think of irritability, declining libido, weight gain, aging skin and hair, depression and anxiety. It is important not to blame everything on menopause.

Some symptoms may also be related to a particular life-stage rather than hormones. The classic example of this is the "empty nest" syndrome, which many women have to face in their late forties or early fifties when children leave home. You keep on worrying about your children, but you may no longer have daily contact with them. It seems a cruel twist of fate that at the same time Nature is taking away your fertility and preventing you from having any more children, the children you do have are leaving home. Trying to explain away these powerful and legitimate feelings in terms of falling hormone levels is to dismiss an important part of many women's experience of motherhood.

At the same time, there may be elderly parents to cope with, too. Few things are more depressing than having to watch a much-loved parent in the final stages of illness. In many cases, parent and daughter swap roles. Women end up being parents to their own parents and taking responsibility for running their lives.

Unfortunately, if a woman of 45 or so goes to her doctor with any of the above symptoms, her problems will immediately be put down to "hormones" and HRT will be offered, even when her periods are still very regular.

Psychological changes

Volatile hormones have a powerful impact on the way we feel, but it's important to remember that they can come into play at any time throughout life and not only at menopause. Just ask any woman who has suffered pre-menstrual syndrome (PMS) — and that includes most of us at one time or another. In fact, the list of so-called menopausal symptoms bears a remarkable similarity to those associated with PMS. It includes:

• Lack of self-esteem
• Less energy and motivation
• Loss of self-confidence
• Mood swings
• Irritability
• Forgetfulness
• Depression
• Anxiety
• Feelings of losing control
• Feeling unable to cope
• Loss of sex drive
• Feeling close to tears
• Vulnerability
• Lack of concentration

These negative feelings can be caused by a hormonal imbalance that may be experienced at any time from your first period on. But as menopause approaches, women who suffer from PMS may find their symptoms getting much worse. Others who have never had PMS can suddenly experience it for the first time.

For other women nearing menopause, the link between hormones and low mood is less direct — some emotional changes may simply be caused by sleep disrupted by night sweats. Experiencing just a few nights of broken sleep is enough to push even a well-balanced woman to the brink of depression. Alternatively, the cause could be that universal problem, stress. But one thing is sure. There is nothing specifically "menopausal" about them at all. This reminds me of one patient who came to me having suffered several of these symptoms quite severely all her life. When she was young she was told that everything would be all right once she had babies. After that, she was told that things would sort themselves out once she was over menopause...

There is of course an entire industry devoted to convincing middle-aged women that they are suffering these symptoms because of menopause, and that taking HRT to replenish their hormones is the best solution to the problem. They may also be prescribed antidepressants and tranquilizers by their doctors, which are potentially addictive and rarely beneficial. The correct way to look at these psychological symptoms is as a continuation of hormonal imbalance, not as something directly caused by menopause. And the correct way to cope with them is to restore the proper balance of mind as well as body through the natural measures described in this book.

What causes hot flashes?

Nobody knows quite what causes the sweating that is the most common symptom of menopause. One theory suggests that it is falling levels of estrogen while another says that the higher levels of FSH are to blame. Whatever the trigger, the immediate effect is the same, because both hot flashes and night sweats are vasomotor symptoms, resulting from changes in the size of the blood vessel designed to control the body's temperature. Blood vessels dilate, or get larger, so that they can allow more blood to flow through and cool you down. It is this automatic reaction that makes you sweat on a hot day.

Hot flashes start as a feeling of heat in the face, neck, or body, which can spread up or down. They can be experienced in different ways. In some cases women may have no outward signs of redness or sweating at all; in others, they may sweat profusely and become extremely red in the face. Some women react with palpitations, others just experience a general increase in body temperature as if somebody has turned up the thermostat. Some flashes last just a few seconds, others for as long as 30 minutes. Afterwards, many women feel cold and shivery, and after taking off layers of clothes, want to put them back on again. The impact of the flashes varies too. Women who only have a few each day can dismiss them as an inconvenience but those who experience four or five an hour may find that their quality of their life is so affected that they feel embarrassed to go out.

Night sweats are basically the same as hot flashes – they just happen at a different time of day. A woman may wake up to find herself drenched in sweat and need to dry herself and change her clothes. As the night sweats are constantly waking her, her pattern of sleep becomes disturbed, resulting in tiredness, depression and irritability. Most of us would feel like this if we were woken up sporadically throughout the night!

Vaginal discomfort

As the level of estrogen falls, the walls of the vagina become thinner and blood flow is restricted, causing a lack of lubrication. Doctors describe this as vaginal "atrophy," which actually means "wasting away" or "becoming useless." It's an unpleasant term, guaranteed to make any woman feel she is about to become a dried-up husk. Luckily this is less likely to occur if you stay sexually active – it's a simple case of "use it or lose it."

Although the vagina does not expand after menopause to the extent it did before, it is still large enough to accommodate an erect penis. Dryness is the main problem, which is where regular sex or masturbation helps. Sexual activity stimulates the blood flow into the vaginal area, reducing dryness, while the muscle contractions that take place during orgasm promote the health of the vagina, helping to keep it elastic.

Your waterworks are also affected by these changes. The walls lining the bladder and urethra (the tube linking the bladder to the outside) shrink, becoming thinner and drier and more prone to bacterial infections like cystitis, especially if they crack and split. You may feel the need to urinate more frequently or find you leak a bit when you sneeze, cough or laugh. The good news is that there are plenty of natural ways to deal with these symptoms, as you will see later on.

CHAPTER 3

What Is Hormone Replacement Therapy (HRT)?

From listening to some enthusiasts, you could easily start to believe that HRT is a wonder-drug with the power to delay aging, increase sex drive, boost memory and stave off osteoporosis as well as eliminating menopausal symptoms such as hot flashes and night sweats. But how do these claims stand up to examination?

Why HRT began

The argument often given for the fact that we "need" HRT is that women are not designed to live past the menopause. Nature intended us to expire when our fertile life is over, the thinking goes, and it is only because of the quality of life in the Western world that we live on for another 30–50 years or more, and therefore need medical help. This reasoning is supposedly supported by the fact that in other species of mammal the female dies at the end of her fertile years, so the human menopause is obviously an aberration. But research shows that many mammals cease producing offspring well before the end of life. In the mammals that have been studied, it seems that the females did not stop having cycles but they did stop producing offspring in their middle age, well before the end of their natural life span. So in fact women are not unique in having another stage of life after their child-bearing years.[1]

These days, women can live another 30 to 50 years past the menopause. Yes, life expectancy was shorter centuries ago, and especially for women, but not because they could not exist without HRT. The statistics are skewed because many women died in childbirth. Exclude these and you will find that many women enjoyed a healthy old age without HRT. Indeed, examinations carried out on the 18th-century remains of a number of women discovered beneath a London church revealed not only that some had died in their 80s, but also that their bone density was better than that of pre-menopausal women today.

Many advocates of HRT also ignore the positive changes this new phase of life can bring. Anthropologists have wondered why men remain fertile until they die while women do not. The conclusion is that there must be an evolutionary advantage or nature would not have created this design. By looking at other cultures such as hunter-gatherer societies,[2] anthropologists have realized that older women have important functions, teaching, preparing food and supporting younger women who are having babies. They become "wise women" and respected elders once childbearing has finished.

In the West, however, the menopause has often been seen in a very negative light. So it is not surprising that in the 1930s, scientists decided that if estrogen drops at the menopause, it should be replaced – by hormone replacement therapy. HRT was originally called estrogen replacement therapy because only estrogen was given, first as injections and from 1938, as implants – pellets of estrogen embedded in the skin.

Neither was very convenient or popular so HRT remained a minority interest until 1966, when gynecologist Robert Wilson wrote a book extolling the virtues of estrogen replacement for women at the menopause. He talked about the "living decay" of the menopause and argued that without estrogen, menopausal women were castrates – the equivalent of eunuchs. Unstable estrogen-starved women, he postulated, were a misery to themselves and everyone else, causing, at worst, alcoholism, drug addiction and broken homes. Contrast this with the state brought about by HRT, an anti-aging treatment which would not only abolish all the symptoms of the menopause, but also keep us, so the title of his book promised, "Feminine Forever."

Unfortunately, it soon became clear that estrogen on its own could increase the risk of cancer of the uterus and breasts.[3] Estrogen builds up the lining of the uterus ready to receive a fertilized egg and without the other main female hormone, progesterone, to trigger bleeding, cell mutations were taking place. When research studies appeared to show that this risk could be up to seven times higher for uterine cancer, there was panic.[4] The risk was too great. Scientists realized that they had to add the other female hormone to prevent this unhealthy build-up of the uterine lining. So progestin, the synthetic version of progesterone, was added to HRT. Since then, only women who have had a hysterectomy have been given estrogen alone.

What HRT contains

Although HRT contains the same steroid sex hormones (estrogen and progestin) as the Pill, the two medications are different.

The main contrast between the Pill and HRT lies in the type and amount of estrogens used. While most contraceptive Pills contain a synthetic estrogen called ethinyl estradiol, many of the estrogens

continued

used in HRT are referred to as "natural." That does not always mean what you might think. In this instance, it usually means that they are chemical equivalents of the hormones produced by the ovaries.

These "natural" estrogens include 17beta-estradiol, estrone, estriol and estrogen conjugates such as estrone sulphate. Other forms, which are esters (organic acid combined with alcohol) of natural estrogens, are estradiol valerate, estradiol cypionate, estradiol phenyl propionate and estradiol benzoate. The conjugated estrogens that are made from the urine of a pregnant mare are also classed as "natural" and contain various different estrogens, a number of which are not natural to humans. These equine estrogens have a different chemical structure from our own estrogens and the body will never have encountered anything like this before. They may be natural to a horse but they are not natural for women.

Some women stopped taking HRT when disturbing reports appeared in the media about its production. In 1995, a representative of the World Society for the Protection of Animals (WSPA) took part in an inspection of 32 farms in Canada that were contracted to supply mare's urine. The following passage is taken from WSPA's report, published in 1996.

"... [A]fter mares have become pregnant, they are brought into barns and housed in individual stalls. A harness-type device... is attached to the animals' rear quarters so that their urine can be collected. The horses spend most of the next six months in these stalls while their estrogen-rich urine is collected.

"Often the horses' stalls were too small to allow the animals to lie down comfortably. In nearly all the farms visited, our inspectors saw tethers that were so short that mares were unable to lay their head on the ground... In all but a few farms, water was being restricted... it is suspected that this is practiced in order to ensure that urine has a high concentration of estrogen."

Most of the HRT preparations contain estradiol, which is the most carcinogenic estrogen, but some contain estrogen in the form of estrone or estriol. In the U.S., healthcare practitioners have access to special pharmacies ("compounding" pharmacies) that can make up any combination and strength of estrogens as required, so treatment can be tailored to suit the individual.

The different kinds of HRT

There are now many different HRT preparations on the market. It is available as patches, gels, vaginal suppositories and creams, implants and tablets and can be taken in a variety of different ways, which result in a period every month, a period every three months, or in theory, no period at all. However, despite the fact that there is plenty of choice, almost four out of 10 women who start taking HRT stop within eight months.

TABLETS

Pills are the most common way of taking HRT, as they are the easiest. Most women take a combination of estrogen and progestin tablets (known as "combined" or "opposed" HRT) to prevent the uterine lining from building up. Only women who have had a hysterectomy are given estrogen continuously, without taking progestin for part of the month (so even if you opt for an HRT patch, implant or gel, you will often end up taking progestin by mouth).

There is a major disadvantage to taking HRT orally, however. All hormones taken by mouth have to be processed by the liver and intestines. This means that the dose has to be higher (about 20 times greater than if the estrogen goes through the skin) because the intestines and liver try to de-activate it. One of the major roles of the liver is to metabolize and neutralize sex hormones, so this organ is just doing what it is supposed to do. To try to overcome this process and get estrogen into the blood, more has to be given.

When this high concentration of estrogen is digested, enormous metabolic changes take place in the liver and the intestinal wall. The result can be an increased risk of gallstones and a rise in the level of fats in the blood, leading to a greater risk of clotting. This activity in the liver also affects the structure of the hormones, and in some cases no substance reaches the circulation unaltered.

It is possible, therefore, that this rise in blood fats and increased risk of clotting means that the likelihood of heart disease could be greater with tablets than with other forms of HRT.[5] As a result, many specialists suggest that it could be better to deliver estrogens via the skin than by mouth. This is closer to the way in which our own hormones work.

One of the advantages of taking HRT in tablet form is that it is easier to manipulate bleeding. Most combined HRT tablets protect the uterus by triggering a monthly period that prevents an unhealthy build-up of the uterine lining. But for many women one of the blessings of the menopause is freedom from periods, so the idea of resuming their periods and perhaps continuing them into their 80s if they stay on HRT is not appealing. So varieties of HRT have been developed which limit bleeding to once every three months or prevent it altogether. This restricted bleed HRT can help women who experience severe PMS-like symptoms as a result of taking progestin. Up to 20 percent of women on combined HRT experience side-effects caused by progestin. These can include bloating, depression, breast tenderness, mood swings, weight gain and irritability – in fact, all the symptoms usually associated with PMS.

The main types of HRT tablet are:

Estrogen-only

Women who have had a hysterectomy do not need progestin because they are no longer at risk of cancer of the uterine lining (endometrial cancer). They take estrogen tablets every day. One of the newer practices is that some women who have not had a hysterectomy are also given estrogen-only tablets and they are checked every few months with a scan by their gynecologist to make sure the uterine lining is not building up.

Monthly bleed

These are called sequential combined HRT. Estrogen tablets are taken for two weeks and tablets containing both estrogen and progestin for the next two weeks. With some preparations there is a seven-day break, with others the estrogen tablets are started again right away.

Quarterly bleed

Estrogen is taken continuously for three months and progestin is added at the end of that time to induce a period.

No bleed

No-bleed (continuous combined) HRT is designed for women who are at least one year past menopause. This low dose, period-free HRT contains a daily dose of estrogen and progestin in one tablet. The balance between the hormones prevents thickening of the uterine lining, so there is no monthly period – in theory anyway, but breakthrough bleeding is common. Up to 50 percent of women experience some bleeding on "no-bleed" HRT even if they take it correctly. The cause is not certain,[6] but if bleeding persists then it needs to be investigated or the HRT preparation changed. Giving progestin and estrogen separately, rather than combining them in a single tablet, sometimes stops breakthrough bleeding, but then PMS-like symptoms can be stronger.

Tibolone, a synthetic steroid compound, which has a weak hormonal action, is another no-bleed medication available for post-menopausal women. It has some of the characteristics of estrogen and progestin plus androgenic, or "male" hormone qualities. There seems to be less spotting and breakthrough bleeding with this preparation because it does not stimulate the uterine lining. But because of its androgenic properties, one of its side-effects can be increased facial hair.

PATCHES

Although patches have the advantage of delivering hormones directly and bypassing the liver, some women find them uncomfortable to use because they can cause irritation. The patch is worn below the waist (the hip and thigh are popular sites) and estrogen enters the body through the skin.

Estrogen patches

Most patches contain estrogen only, so unless you have had a hysterectomy, you will need to take progestin tablets for the next 12–14 days of the second half of the cycle to protect your uterus. Originally, the estrogen was released through a small reservoir on the reverse of the patch. In newer patches it forms part of the adhesive layer and the patch can be cut to size to vary the dose.

Combined patches

It is possible to use patches containing progestin as an alternative to taking it by mouth. Estrogen patches are used for the first two weeks, followed by combined estrogen and progestin patches for the next fortnight. Combined patches should not be cut or altered in any way as the dose is carefully regulated to cause the bleed that protects the uterine lining.

IMPLANTS

Also called subcutaneous HRT, these are pellets inserted beneath the skin, usually in the lower abdomen, by your doctor. Most implants contain six months' supply of estrogen, although in some cases testosterone implants are also given to help women with low libido. (Possible side-effects include a deepening voice, growth of facial hair and loss of hair on the head, however, so it is definitely better to tackle this problem using natural remedies – see page 116.)

Implants have a number of advantages. As they are not ingested, the hormones bypass the liver and go directly into the bloodstream, which means that the dose can be lower but just as effective. Many women find them convenient, because once an implant is inserted, you can forget about it. Wrong doses cannot be easily changed, however, and implants can be difficult to remove if you decide to stop HRT. And unless you have had a hysterectomy, you will still need to take progestin tablets in addition to your estrogen implant to induce a monthly bleed. Worryingly, implants have often been inserted during a hysterectomy without the woman knowing about it until later.

More alarming is the fact that some women using implants develop a form of estrogen-dependency and require ever larger amounts for the HRT to work effectively. Symptoms associated with the menopause seem to recur at shorter and shorter intervals so the implants have to be replaced much more frequently. When their hormone levels are tested, these women often have very high levels of estrogen, yet they still complain of menopausal symptoms such as hot flashes. No one knows quite why this happens. One theory is that in women with implants the body is not able to use the estrogen properly. Another is that the body becomes used to a particular dose and therefore needs ever-increasing amounts to relieve the symptoms. This phenomenon is called tachyphylaxis, and the same thing happens when diamorphine (a type of morphine) is given to relieve pain.[7]

The problems associated with implants prompted investigation by the Food and Drug Administration. The pellets are supposed to dissolve slowly, releasing a controlled amount of hormone and allowing estrogen levels to return to baseline before a new implant is inserted. These safeguards should prevent estrogen rising to unacceptable levels, but it emerged that women were not being monitored properly. One woman was awarded compensation after it was discovered that she had 18 implants in her body that had failed to dissolve.

This accumulation of estrogen means that the end result is very high levels of estradiol circulating around the body, well above the levels normal even for pre-menopausal women, accompanied, ironically, by the return of hot flashes. For women with these high levels of estrogen from repeated use of implants, it can take many years for the excess estrogen to be eliminated from the body once the woman has stopped having the implants.[8]

This has prompted concern about the impact of high estrogen levels on the uterus and breast tissue. One suggestion is that progestin should be given for a while after implants have been removed, and that women should have their uterine lining checked for abnormalities.[9]

NASAL SPRAY

A new delivery system for HRT is an estrogen nasal spray inhaled once a day. Although this is an easy method of taking HRT, you are advised not to blow your nose within 15 minutes of sniffing it. (It is not yet known whether sneezing affects its efficacy.) Unless you have had a hysterectomy you will still need to take progestin tablets to prevent the uterine lining from building up, since the spray is an estrogen–only preparation.

GELS

Gels containing estrogen that can be rubbed on to the lower abdomen are useful for women who find that they react to the adhesive in patches. As with the patch, the hormone is absorbed through the skin and the dose of estrogen can be lower because it bypasses the liver. Because the gel contains only estrogen, most women also have to take progestin. A popular regime is to use the gel and then take progestin for 12-14 days once every three months to induce a bleed.

VAGINAL HRT

This type of HRT is designed to help with vaginal discomfort without affecting the rest of the body. It contains enough estrogen to tackle problems such as vaginal itchiness and dryness but too little to help with hot flashes. Because vaginal HRT only contains a small amount of estrogen, it is not usually necessary to take progestin.

Vaginal creams and suppositories are inserted directly into the vagina with an applicator. There are a number of different types containing various kinds of estrogens. Estriol is the least likely to trigger cancer, so I suggest asking for a product based on this type of estrogen (but best of all, try the recommendations on pages 145–147 for the natural approach to vaginal dryness).

The vaginal ring is impregnated with estrogen and inserted high into the vagina where it remains for three months and is then replaced. The ring is normally recommended for women with vaginal dryness or problems with the urinary tract but again, it cannot help with hot flashes. It is recommended that it is not used continuously for more than two years.

SELECTIVE ESTROGEN RECEPTOR MODULATORS (SERMs)

SERMs are one of the latest HRTs on the block. Many women are reluctant to stay on conventional HRT for extended periods because of the risk of breast cancer. Therefore, scientists have been focusing on SERMs, a new generation of designer HRTs that can provide the beneficial effects of estrogen where needed (the bones for example) while avoiding any stimulating effects, and even acting as an "anti-estrogen," in areas where too much estrogen can be dangerous (such as the breast and uterus).

In our bodies there are two kinds of estrogen receptors, alpha and beta. The alpha receptors are located in the uterus, ovaries and breasts and the beta receptors are in the brain, blood vessels, bones, uterus, breasts and ovaries. So you can see that some parts of the body – breasts, uterus and ovaries – have both alpha and beta receptors. SERMs block the alpha receptors in the breasts, uterus and ovaries (which stops excess stimulation) but have a positive, stimulating effect on the beta receptors in the brain, bones and blood vessels. Conventional HRT seems to trigger the activity of both alpha and beta receptors, so causing stimulation of breast and uterine tissue and hence the increased risk of breast and uterine cancer.

Tamoxifen, the drug used to prevent a recurrence of breast cancer, was the first available SERM. Tamoxifen works as an anti-estrogen by blocking the estrogen receptors in the breast. But when picked up by the receptors in the uterus, the tamoxifen can actually increase the risk of uterine cancer because it has a stimulatory effect on the receptors in the uterine lining.

Most drug companies are now working on creating other versions of designer estrogens. One of the newest SERMs on the scene is raloxifene, which has been approved for prevention of osteoporosis, but its full potential is still being investigated. At the moment, possible side-effects include increased clots and even an increase in hot flashes! In other words, it is useless in the treatment of major menopausal symptoms such as hot flashes and night sweats, which are, of course, one of the main reasons why women are attracted to HRT. It is, however, aimed at women who want protection for their bones without running the risk of breast cancer and is offered to women who are at least one year past their last period.

Like conventional HRT, raloxifene has been shown to increase bone mineral density in women after menopause.[10] SERMs can also reduce the risk of spinal fractures in post-menopausal women with osteoporosis.[11] But the question remains, can SERMs reduce fractures in post-menopausal women who have never had a fracture?

Fortunately, there is a natural counterpart to these designer HRTs. Phytoestrogens, such as soy and chickpeas (see page 48), can be thought of as nature's SERMs.[12] They have a weak estrogenic effect that can help to ease menopausal symptoms and, like SERMs, block the alpha receptors in the breasts, uterus and ovaries (which stops excess stimulation) but have a positive, stimulating effect on the beta receptors in the brain, bones and blood vessels.[13]

The side-effects of HRT

The Physician's Desk Reference lists the following as the possible side-effects of HRT (besides uterine cancer):

- undesirable weight gain/loss
- breast tenderness/enlargement
- bloating
- depression
- thrombophlebitis (inflammation of a vein)
- raised blood pressure
- reduced carbohydrate tolerance
- skin rashes
- hair loss
- abdominal cramps
- vaginal candidiasis (thrush)
- jaundice
- vomiting
- cystitis-like problems

Although these conditions are uncomfortable rather than life-threatening, it is often immediate discomfort rather than long-term risk that makes women reconsider their decision to take HRT. Take weight gain, for example. Although there is no research to show that women on HRT gain any more weight than that normally associated with aging, I find that this is one of the greatest concerns expressed by women who come to see me. Their complaints center on the breast enlargement and "sudden" increase in weight – up to 28 pounds – that occur soon after starting HRT, without any changes in their diet. I also see women who are not on HRT and the two groups of women definitely experience different types of weight gain (see page 184).

Headaches and psychological changes – suicidal thoughts and feeling "not there," as if you are watching your life from outside – are other common side-effects. Not surprisingly, women who experience these frequently come to the conclusion that the side-effects are worse than the symptoms HRT is designed to cure.

The long-term health risks

In addition to these immediate problems, there is growing evidence that HRT involves major health risks when taken for a long period of time. Although many women feel perfectly well on HRT, as the years roll on, the likelihood of serious disease increases. The evidence that has recently emerged is even more alarming.

The supposed long-term "benefits" of HRT are also looking more like myths. It may have once seemed that some of the risks associated with HRT were worth taking because of the positive effects it had on the heart and bones, but this is no longer the case. If you take HRT, there are only two benefits you can really hope to attain. The first is that it alleviates hot flashes and night sweats, the second that it maintains bone density for as long as you take it. You may therefore conclude that HRT carries little long-term benefit, only risks such as breast cancer. Not a good trade-off, in my opinion.

WHAT CAN GO WRONG?

BREAST CANCER

Of all the risks associated with taking HRT, this is the one that concerns women the most, and understandably so. It was first suggested as long ago as 1976, when the *New England Journal of Medicine* reported a study linking estrogen in HRT to an increase in breast cancer.[14]

Numerous studies since have confirmed this finding. In 1997, a review of data from more than 40 studies and 60,000 women showed that HRT increases the risk of breast cancer by 35 percent when taken for more than 11 years.[15] In the early part of 2000 two more substantial studies were published, again confirming an increase in the risk of breast cancer for women on HRT. One, from the *Journal of the American Medical Association*, studied over 46,000 women and found a 40 percent increase in breast cancer risk in those taking HRT.[16]

With the evidence stretching back almost 30 years, surely the warning bells should have been ringing loud and clear? But it took until the summer of 2002, when a major research program from the Women's Health Initiative was abandoned, for the dangers of HRT to make a serious impact. The research program, focusing on 27,000 women, was due to run until 2005 but was cancelled after a follow-up survey at five years that showed that the women taking HRT had a 26 percent higher risk of breast cancer, a 41 percent increase in the chance of a stroke and a 29 percent increased heart risk.[17] Some doctors have attempted to console women by saying that even though there is a risk, the breast cancers that develop when women take HRT are easier to treat. Not an argument I would find reassuring!

Scientific evidence shows not only that taking HRT is definitely associated with an increased risk of developing breast cancer but also that the risk is there right from the start; it does not suddenly shoot up after five years of use as has been previously suggested. Obviously the risk is less if you have only been taking HRT for two years rather than five, but it rises by 2.3 percent for each year on medication. It is estimated that a woman on combined HRT increases her risk of breast cancer by approximately 80 percent after 10 years compared to a woman who has never taken it.

The good news is that conversely, the likelihood of developing breast cancer goes down rapidly when women stop taking HRT. You can reduce this risk still further by taking care of your health and making sure that your liver is really healthy, because this is the organ that helps to detoxify hormones (see page 72). Naturally, the health of your liver is especially important if you decide to stay on HRT.

So what exactly is the link between HRT and breast cancer? The immediate cause of the rise in breast cancer is that HRT stimulates breast tissue and makes it thicker. Radiographers and ultrasonographers report that the breasts of women who take HRT are denser and more opaque than women who don't, which could mean that small tumors may be missed.[18] It is also well established that HRT can trigger the development of breast cysts and enlarge existing benign tumors called fibroadenomas.[19] But women taking tibolone (a synthetic steroid compound with weak male and female hormone actions; see page 25) or raloxifene (a SERM; see page 29) rather than conventional HRT do not experience these changes in breast density.[20]

My recommendation to any woman thinking of going on HRT is to have a breast ultrasound scan first (see page 157), or if that is not possible, a mammogram. If this reveals any hint of breast disease or an already increased breast density before you have even started on HRT, try the natural ways to manage the menopause outlined in this book instead. Adding in hormones when there is a pre-existing problem could stimulate cells to change and mutate where they might otherwise have stayed dormant.

UTERINE (ENDOMETRIAL) CANCER

Estrogen's role in the body is to increase cell growth, so it is logical that it could directly affect the parts of a woman's body that are most receptive to it, such as the uterus and breasts. A 1975 study in the *New England Journal of Medicine* showed that women who took estrogen alone had a sevenfold increased risk of developing uterine cancer,[21] and ever since, women who have not had a hysterectomy have been prescribed progestin to protect the uterine lining.

The addition of progestin is designed to cushion the uterus from the stimulating effects of estrogen, preventing a buildup of the uterine lining by encouraging a regular period. Even so, women on combined HRT have more than double the risk of developing uterine cancer compared to women who don't take HRT at all.[22]

THROMBOSIS (CLOTS) AND STROKE

HRT can increase the risk of thrombosis (blood clots) implicated in heart attack and stroke. The risk is especially acute in the first year, when it is twice or three times greater than for women who are not on HRT.[23]

Blood clots that break free can wreak havoc in the heart or brain, and it is known that women who take HRT have a threefold greater risk of stroke.[24] The evidence is so clear now because the long-term Women's Health Initiative research program was abandoned and the 27,000 women involved in the program warned that HRT can cause a 41 percent increased risk of stroke.[25]

The effect of HRT on clots is not surprising because the same link exists between blood clots and the Pill. Although there are differences in dose and the chemical makeup, the Pill and HRT contain essentially the same combination of hormones.

HEART DISEASE

For a long time, HRT was thought to prevent heart disease (see Chapter 10), and this has been one of the main reasons for recommending it. Heart disease rises in women over 50 when protective estrogen levels start to fall, so giving estrogen should decrease the risk, the thinking goes. But rather than lowering the risk of heart disease, new research shows that HRT actually seems to increase it. As a result, the proposed eight-year clinical trial run by the Women's Health Initiative had to be stopped because the evidence was showing that women on HRT had a 29 percent increased risk of heart disease.

GALL BLADDER DISEASE

HRT can also increase the risk of gall bladder disease, caused by increased

Flying, deep vein thrombosis and HRT

Given that HRT can increase the risk of blood clots, what are the implications for women taking it who intend to fly?

The danger is the possibility of deep vein thrombosis (DVT), a blood clot that develops in the calf. It is not dangerous in itself but can be fatal if the clot breaks free and moves into the lungs or heart. Unfortunately, symptoms can occur days or weeks after the flight.

It was originally thought that DVT was part of an "economy class syndrome" caused by hours spent sitting in cramped conditions in a

continued

pressurized cabin, which can have grave consequences for the circulation. As the majority of air travelers are men, you might expect that most of those affected by DVT would be male. But according to the UK Aviation Health Institute, the majority of DVT victims (64 percent) are women.

Two of the risk factors listed for DVT are the Pill and HRT, medications taken by millions of women, which may be why women account for the majority of victims. Some were women in their 20s – women who would not normally have been affected by other risk factors such as heart disease, cancer, varicose veins, recent surgery or age.

If you are on HRT and are planning a long-haul flight, you need to think about whether it would be best to come off it until you return home. The good news is that although the risk of clots rises while you are taking HRT, past use of HRT does not result in an increased risk.[26]

It is important not to rely on taking aspirin to prevent DVT. Contrary to public opinion, this is not considered helpful. Although aspirin is an anti-platelet agent, which disperses the clots that can lead to heart attack, platelets do not play a large part in DVT.[27] (Platelets are disc-shaped cell structures in the blood whose main function is to stem bleeding.) However, there are other precautions you can take. Elastic flight socks seem to be very helpful in preventing DVT, along with self-help measures such as exercising your legs, drinking plenty of water and avoiding alcohol. Other natural ways to help prevent DVT would be to take the herb ginkgo biloba, which increases blood flow by regulating the tone and elasticity of blood vessels. Bromelain, a derivative of pineapple, breaks down small clots while pycnogenol, a pine bark supplement, reduces clotting and reinforces the capillary walls.

levels of estrogen in the system that lead to metabolic changes in the liver.[28] Women taking HRT are three times more likely to develop gallstones and the risk rises the longer a woman takes HRT.

OVARIAN CANCER

Because there is a link between HRT and breast cancer, questions have also been asked about whether it could also increase the risk of another cancer linked to female hormones, ovarian cancer. Currently the evidence seems to show that women taking HRT could be at greater risk. Although more research is needed, it seems sensible to avoid HRT if you have a family history of ovarian cancer and to manage menopause naturally instead.[29]

The "long-term benefits" of HRT: sifting the evidence

If the benefits of any medication you are given do not outweigh the risks, it is not worth taking the drug. Over the years, HRT has been pushed by the media and enthusiastic doctors as the solution to all menopausal problems. It is supposed to give women renewed energy, increased libido and a wide range of health benefits with very little risk. It now seems that the long-term risks of HRT are not as "little" as was first thought, but what about the long-term benefits? After all, in addition to its role in controlling hot flashes and night sweats, it has been suggested that HRT could help to prevent heart disease, osteoporosis, Alzheimer's disease and colon cancer, to name just a few.

In an attempt to sift through the evidence, a report called "The International Position Paper on Women's Health and Menopause," written by 28 doctors and scientists, was published in 2002. They reviewed all the studies on HRT and concluded that "over the past few years, all these things we've thought about the wonders of hormone replacement may not be holding up under scrutiny." Examples include the finding that rather than giving protection from heart attack and strokes, HRT may increase the risk, and the revelation that no large randomized controlled trials had ever been conducted to see whether HRT reduces fractures.

An additional concern centers on the accuracy of the claims for HRT. The editors of a number of medical journals have warned drug companies to take a back seat in clinical trials. In 2002 *The Lancet* ran an editorial entitled "Just how tainted has medicine become?"[30] There are concerns that financial interests are skewing the results of drug trials, that in some cases the benefits of drugs have been hyped in research papers, and that side-effects have been disguised. Many influential medical journals have said that unless clinical trials are proved to be independent, they will not publish the results.

What is clear is that only now, after HRT has been used in different forms since the 1930s, are the long-term effects being made widely known and that in effect for the last 70 or so years, women have been involved in one huge experiment. My advice is definitely to try the natural approach first for this natural stage in your life.

WHAT'S THE EVIDENCE FOR HRT AND ...

... OSTEOPOROSIS?

One of the main reasons women take HRT is that that they think it will protect their bones. Such is their fear of osteoporosis that women are willing to take powerful hormones to try to prevent something that may never happen – even though perfectly benign measures such as diet and exercise can be just as effective.

Of course, there is one question that women desperately want answered: does HRT prevent fractures? Almost all the clinical trials have focused on the impact of HRT on bone mineral density, the argument being that because bone density increases when women take HRT, then HRT must prevent fractures. But the fact is that increasing bone density and preventing fractures are two very different things. For example, although calcium taken with vitamin D reduces the risk of fractures, it has little or no effect on bone density.[31] And interestingly, there is a condition called osteopetrosis, which people are born with. Their bones are very dense but brittle and tend to fracture, so a good bone density does not necessarily mean that fractures will be prevented.

There has only been one randomized clinical trial that concentrated solely on HRT and fracture reduction,[32] and in that one trial, the use of HRT did not show any statistically significant reduction in the number of broken bones. The large Women's Health Initiative, which was designed to focus on the effects of HRT on cardiovascular disease,[33] did show, however, that HRT reduced the risk of hip fractures by 35 percent and vertebral fractures by 34 percent.

In any case, the increase in bone density brought about by HRT is only temporary because when women stop taking HRT, they often experience a rapid decline in bone density.[34] Indeed, one study of elderly women who had taken HRT when they were younger showed that by the time they had reached the age of 75 to 80 (when fractures are most common), their bone density was only marginally higher than that of women who had never taken HRT.

The belief that HRT can protect the bones seems even more spurious when you consider that the Food and Drug Administration has withdrawn approval for the use of the oldest and most popular form of HRT, conjugated equine estrogen (from pregnant mares' urine), as a treatment for osteoporosis. Furthermore, at a meeting of the American Association of Clinical Endocrinologists in 2001, delegates were reminded that "estrogen is not approved for the treatment of osteoporosis." This followed results from two large clinical trials suggesting that although HRT increases bone density, it does not reduce the incidence of fractures. Even more worryingly, in one of these trials women taking HRT had more fractures than women on dummy pills.[35]

All the evidence indicates that even if you have osteoporosis, there are more effective treatments than HRT (see page 91) and that for 50-year-old women who do not have osteoporosis "the benefits of long-term treatment with estrogen to prevent bone loss and fractures may not exceed the risks."[36] So what's the bottom line? Don't take HRT to prevent fractures because the risks aren't worth it.

... Alzheimer's and memory loss?

Although it was once thought that estrogen would slow the progression of Alzheimer's disease, HRT appears to be of no benefit. Indeed, there is some concern that it could speed it up.[37] Trials on HRT and memory loss are still being carried out, but in the meantime, if you want to avoid taking hormones, there are several natural alternatives that may help (see page 138).

... depression?

HRT can certainly improve symptoms of depression, mood swings and well-being, but only where these are triggered by hot flashes, night sweats and sleep disturbances.[38] Studies show that women who do not have hot flashes and night sweats who take HRT report no improved quality of life in terms of their energy, mental health and physical activity. In some cases, their energy levels and the amount of exercise they take are actually lower than they are in women who are not on HRT.

... urinary incontinence?

Contrary to popular belief, HRT does not help urinary incontinence. In fact, it has been shown to make the problem worse.[39] In one study, more improvement was found in women taking dummy pills than in those on HRT, and incontinence increased in 39 percent of women on HRT, compared to 27 percent of the women taking the placebo. The deterioration associated with HRT was seen after only four months of taking it and was apparent for both urge and stress incontinence.

... colon cancer?

Research is still showing that HRT has a protective effect against colon cancer (by 37 percent),[40] but we now know that diet can have a significant effect on preventing this type of cancer too. In my opinion it is not worth risking breast cancer to prevent colon cancer.

Your questions answered

HOW WILL I KNOW WHEN I'VE REACHED THE MENOPAUSE IF I'M TAKING HRT?

The answer is that you won't, until you stop taking it. Menopause is usually confirmed when you have not had a period for 12 consecutive months. If you start HRT before your periods stop, you will not know when your periods come to a natural end because you will continue to have a monthly bleed.

CAN I GET PREGNANT WHILE TAKING HRT?

Yes, because HRT does not act as a contraceptive. If you start HRT before your periods stop, you could still be ovulating. To be safe from pregnancy, you should continue taking precautions until you have two years without a period if you are under 50, one year if you are over 50. The dilemma is that starting HRT while you still have periods throws the calculation out, because you will not know when menopause occurs.

HOW SHOULD I COME OFF HRT?

Often women are simply told to stop straight away, but unfortunately this can lead to rebound effects, which are linked to estrogen withdrawal. It is well known that hot flashes are linked to estrogen withdrawal and not just low estrogen levels.[41] This means that if you stop HRT suddenly, you can end up with worse hot flashes than the ones that made you take HRT in the first place. The best way to avoid this is to wean yourself off HRT. Ask your doctor for a lower dose and aim to come off completely in three months. At the same time, start following the recommendations in this book to cushion the withdrawal effects (see page 108).

If you cannot reduce the dose of the HRT, you could switch to a patch. Because the patch delivers estrogen through the skin and does not have to be broken down by the liver first, you can get by with a lower dose than if it is taken by mouth. Alternatively, you could use an estrogen gel, rubbing in smaller amounts of estrogen each time. Remember, though, that the dosage of the progestin must not be altered if you are on a type of HRT that stimulates a withdrawal bleed. It is important that this happens each month until you come off HRT entirely.

I WANT TO TAKE HRT BUT I'M WORRIED ABOUT BREAST CANCER. IS THERE ANY TEST I CAN HAVE TO MAKE THAT DECISION EASIER?

Obviously my recommendation is to try the natural approach first, but if you decide to take HRT I would suggest that you begin by having an ultrasound scan or a mammogram. This should detect any abnormalities in your breasts or breast thickening that may be stimulated by the estrogen in HRT, and help you avoid any possible problems.

IF I HAVE HAD BREAST CANCER SHOULD I USE HRT?

My answer to this would be a definite no. Given the scientific evidence, in my opinion it is just not worth the risk. I have seen some women who have had an estrogen-dependent cancer and been given Tamoxifen, an anti-estrogen, to prevent a recurrence. But one of the side-effects of Tamoxifen is hot flashes – and they were then given HRT for the hot flashes!

IF I'VE GOT FIBROIDS/ENDOMETRIOSIS SHOULD I USE HRT?

Both of these conditions are sensitive to estrogen, and as women reach menopause these conditions actually start to sort themselves out because estrogen levels are naturally declining. Adding HRT to the equation means that these conditions can be stimulated to grow.

One woman came to see me because her fibroid, which had been perfectly manageable, had grown to an enormous size when she began taking HRT. She now has no choice but to have a hysterectomy because the fibroid has become so large.

DOES HRT DELAY MENOPAUSE?

No, HRT does not stop the clock. If a woman goes on HRT before her periods stop, and she then comes off it at the age of 60, for example, then her periods will not return. So HRT does not prolong fertility. But remember that it is possible you could still become pregnant if you were still having periods when you started taking it.

CHAPTER 4

"Natural" Progesterone

The use of "natural" progesterone instead of conventional HRT has given rise to some of the most heated but interesting discussions and debates. Not long ago natural progesterone was considered by many to be far superior to conventional HRT and a safe form of self-treatment that would help every symptom of menopause. Why?

The thinking behind it is that the world is suffering from an excess of estrogen. Industry constantly bombards us with xenoestrogens (see page 164), artificial versions of estrogen often derived from petrochemicals and found in packaging, plastics, foods and pesticides. An increasing number of disturbing developments are blamed on these chemicals and they are believed to have a devastating effect on fertility, reproduction and health for both humans and animals. In the West, it is reckoned that men's sperm counts may have dropped by 50 percent in the last 10 years. Other studies have linked these xenoestrogens to the increase in breast and testicular cancers and to other estrogen-dependent conditions such as endometriosis and fibroids.

An additional problem for women in midlife is that in the years before menopause, many have periods without ovulating. If ovulation is absent, a woman will not produce progesterone in that cycle and will have a dominance of estrogen. So it seemed logical that taking progesterone would counteract all this unwanted estrogen.

In reality, however, this is hardly a sensible approach. While I certainly believe that our lifestyles and environment have a profound effect on our health, I do not believe that the answer is to introduce ever more hormones into our bodies. It is much better to take more care over our nutrition, which has such an impact on the body's biochemical processes, and to take steps to control the xenoestrogens coming in from outside (see page 164).

Just how "natural" is progesterone anyway?

Progesterone has a long history. It was originally obtained from sows' ovaries, but by the late 1930s it could be synthesized from placentas in large amounts. So placentas were quick-frozen after delivery for later extraction of progesterone.

After a number of years a way was found of converting a substance called diosgenin from the wild yam (Dioscorea villosa) into progesterone. This diosgenin became the starting point in the chemical manufacturing process of progesterone, which was converted to the synthetic progestin first used in birth control pills and later in HRT. Because progesterone is a fat-soluble compound, it is usually ineffective when taken by mouth since it is first metabolized by the liver and never gets into the bloodstream in sufficient amounts. This led to progesterone being given intramuscularly by injection and also as a suppository inserted into the vagina or rectum. It is now available in the form of cream to rub on the surface of the skin and is sold over the counter as a cosmetic.

This "natural" progesterone is often thought of as an extract of wild yam. In fact, progesterone itself is not found in wild yam. It is synthesized from the plant by a number of chemical steps, which means it is not "natural" at all. The assumption was that if you ate wild yam or put it on your skin, your body could convert it into the biologically active human hormone progesterone. This is simply not true. While progesterone can be synthesized from diosgenin, it can only be done by a chemist in a laboratory. The human body is just not capable of synthesizing progesterone from a substance such as wild yam (and in fact these progesterone creams do not contain any wild yam at all). Progesterone is called "natural" progesterone because it is chemically identical to the progesterone produced by humans and to differentiate it from the synthetic progestin used in HRT.

It is important to be aware that progesterone creams contain a powerful pharmaceutical hormone that is made in a laboratory. The Food and Drug Administration won't allow the manufacturers of such creams to make medicinal claims, so they are sold as cosmetics (like a moisturizer), not as hormone replacements. Wild yam has a respectable reputation as a herbal treatment for menstrual problems. For centuries, herbalists have used wild yam in a tincture form and it has traditionally been used as an anti-spasmodic and anti-inflammatory herb. Since the essence of herbal medicine is that all the ingredients contribute to the overall therapeutic effect, diosgenin alone is unlikely to be responsible for the wild yam's beneficial qualities. Herbs work because they contain a host of substances − active substances, balancing substances and substances that cope with any side-effects of the active substances. They are holistic and truly "natural." But the "natural" progesterone that is being hyped is no more "natural" than a number of the plant-based estrogen preparations that form the basis of some HRT drugs.

As you can see, my main concern is that women have been duped into thinking they are buying a natural herbal remedy containing wild yam. Let me reiterate: they are not. They are buying hormone replacement – just a different hormone (progesterone instead of the usual HRT combination of a form of estrogen plus progestin). The theory behind it is the same as the theory behind conventional HRT – that menopausal women are suffering from a hormone deficiency disorder, a modern complaint that has arisen because we are now living way beyond our reproductive years.

My approach is quite different, and truly natural, as it teaches your body to balance your hormones using nutrition and herbs. This holistic approach covers every part of your lifestyle. It works by encouraging your body to find its natural hormone balance, which will promote bone health and relieve a whole host of other symptoms at the same time. You change your diet, you add food supplements (substances you would normally eat but perhaps need in more concentrated forms for a while) so your digestion improves, increasing your ability to absorb nutrients. Herbal medicine, acupuncture and homeopathy are used where appropriate. The result is good health and balanced hormones. Isn't this the best way forward?

Some unanswered questions

I have a number of questions to address to the pro-natural progesterone camp: How much should a woman take? Will she end up with too much progesterone (as I have seen in some women)? When should she stop taking it? Dr. John Lee, one of the foremost advocates of progesterone, suggests that women take it until they reach the age of 85, after which they should be reassessed. That's a long time to take any drug.

One of my other concerns is that a number of women I have seen have been experimenting on their own and manipulating the HRT given to them by their doctors. If they are on an HRT that is supposed to give a monthly bleed, part of the treatment contains progestin in order to shed the uterine lining. Unfortunately, many women experience side-effects from the progestin which can include bloating, depression, breast tenderness, mood swings, weight gain and irritability – hence the temptation to use progesterone cream instead, which does not cause these symptoms.

Unfortunately, it seems that the amount absorbed from "natural" progesterone cream is not enough to protect the uterine lining from the thickening effects of the estrogen.[1] If you have been using a progesterone cream plus estrogen then you should see your doctor to have an ultrasound scan to make sure that the uterine lining has not built up excessively (endometrial hyperplasia). The risk if left is that the cells could become cancerous. Oral micronized (ground into tiny particles) progesterone tablets are available by prescription and they do seem to protect the uterine lining from the stimulating effect of estrogen.[2]

The claims made for progesterone

The hope has been that progesterone could protect the bones, while avoiding any unwanted effects on the breasts. Sadly, however, the evidence does not stand up to scrutiny.

PROGESTERONE AND OSTEOPOROSIS

One claim that has been made for progesterone is that it can combat osteoporosis, but in a study conducted by Dr. John Lee, women not only used progesterone cream but changed their diet, took supplements, and began an exercise program too. Some may even have been taking estrogen. I would suggest that the consequent improvement in their bones could well be caused by these other factors.

Although there are a number of other studies under way comparing the effect of progesterone cream on osteoporosis with that of a placebo (dummy) cream, it will be a number of years before we know the results. Right now, nobody knows whether progesterone has any valuable effect on the bones, and I am concerned that women using the cream are being treated as guinea pigs.

To be sure, studies may eventually show that progesterone is beneficial, but for the time being, remember this: whatever the label says, progesterone cream is not a natural product, and by adding chemicals to your body on a daily basis you may well be taking an unacceptable risk. Do you actually need more progesterone? Do you need additional estrogen, for that matter?

Adding a hormone (which is just another form of drug) to the body will never address the fundamental cause of fragile bones. Even if progesterone is shown to increase bone density, as soon as you stop using the cream that benefit may stop. And if you have relied on extra hormones rather than diet and exercise to protect your bones, your body as a whole will be no healthier.

PROGESTERONE AND BREAST CANCER

Although it has been suggested that progesterone can protect against breast cancer, it actually has a direct effect on breast growth. In fact, studies are showing that higher levels of progesterone may actually be a risk factor for breast cancer.[3]

You may find this surprising, because while too much estrogen can trigger cancer of the uterus, progesterone can protect against its effects. The breasts and the uterus have receptors for both the female hormones, estrogen and progesterone, and there seems no reason why a difference in location should affect their function. However, it has been shown that progesterone receptors in the breast do respond differently than those in the uterus.[4]

What this comes down to is that if you take extra progesterone, you could increase your risk of breast cancer. If you take estrogen on its own, you may increase your risk of both uterine and breast cancer.

★

Progesterone v. progestin

It's easy to think that these are two words for the same thing, but they're not. Although progesterone and progestin have some similarities, in other respects they are very different.

Progesterone is produced by the ovaries. As soon as the egg has been released, the ruptured ovarian follicle develops into what is called the corpus luteum, which produces progesterone. As progesterone levels rise, the body temperature goes up too (a sign of ovulation) ready to "incubate" the fertilized egg. If you are pregnant, progesterone continues to rise. If you are not, progesterone (and estrogen) levels fall and you have a period. Progesterone is the most important female hormone during the second half of the cycle and is absolutely necessary to maintain a pregnancy. If a woman is not producing sufficient progesterone when the egg is fertilized, she could miscarry.

Progestin is a synthetic hormone used in both the Pill and combined HRT, where it prevents the uterine lining from building up excessively. Two types of progestin are included in HRT preparations. The first group (such as dydrogesterone and medroxyprogesterone) is based on progesterone and the second (such as norethisterone) is derived from testosterone. Progestins that are similar to progesterone may cause enlargement of the breasts, while those similar to testosterone can stimulate the growth of facial hair.

So why not take progesterone, you may ask? Unfortunately, the natural hormone is usually ineffective when taken by mouth. Because it is a fat-soluble compound, it is changed by the liver and rarely reaches the bloodstream in sufficient amounts. Progestin, on the other hand, is

continued

not affected by the liver and has the added convenience that the dose can be easily controlled.

Although progestin is able to fulfill many of progesterone's functions, the body has difficulty "recognizing" and coping with it because it is not a natural hormone, hence the well-known side-effects such as mood swings, depression and so on. Furthermore, recent research published in the *International Journal of Cancer* shows that progestins can increase the growth of new blood vessels that will allow a tumor to develop.[6]

It was almost 20 years before it was realized that estrogen used on its own dramatically increased the risk of endometrial cancer. Are we going to wait another 20 years for the progesterone time-bomb to explode?

CHAPTER 5

Your Diet at Menopause

What you eat at menopause is the key to your health. Good nutrition enables your body to adjust to the changes automatically and keep your hormones in balance, avoiding and preventing disease. Give your body natural foods that it can digest easily and use to maximum benefit, and it will have everything you need to respond to the different stages of your life.

Let's start by exploding a myth. There are no such things as "health foods" or "healthy foods." That is just marketing hype. I have always found it strange that we have "health food" stores. Does that mean the others are "ill health food" stores and if so, why would people choose to eat food that is going to make them ill? Survival is your body's top priority and it will use whatever nourishment you give it to try to keep healthy. However, you can make this job much harder by providing poor-quality food and drink that will eventually lead to ill health. Or you can make it much easier by providing a quality diet that will keep you feeling fit and well.

If you can keep your body in balance, you will allow your own hormones to work as efficiently as possible, using the estrogen available from the adrenal glands and fat cells. In this way you have a much better chance of reducing the symptoms of menopause to a minimum and even avoiding them altogether.

Changing for the better

Eating is a time for sharing and socializing, so the recommendations outlined in this section are meant to encourage an enjoyable, pleasurable and healthy way of eating. This is not a diet that you follow for a while and then abandon in favor of a former unhealthy eating pattern. It is easy to follow, full of variety, and importantly, very tasty. I know this because this is the way I eat, too.

Of course there may be occasions when it is not possible to follow the guide-lines – when you are out to dinner or on vacation for instance – but so long as your basic diet is good, a few deviations from it will not make much difference. Remember this is not a strict regime but a plan for making improvements in your eating pattern to enhance your health and well-being. Above all, it is to be enjoyed.

Some changes are fairly easy to make. These include adding fresh, tasty foods and making better choices – opting for organic free-range eggs instead of factory ones or pure diluted fruit juice instead of cola or other soft drinks, for example. Others, such as giving up coffee, tea and sugary snacks, may be harder. Don't be put off because you think altering your eating habits sounds difficult. Try taking one step at a time. You'll be pleasantly surprised at how well you can adapt to changes if you make them gradually. And even if you are not able to make all the changes suggested, it is worth doing what you can.

I have split this section into what to eat and what not to eat. The aim is to help you to make any changes that may be necessary by explaining how different foods and drinks affect your body. Once you understand these effects, you can take control of your health. You will know what and when to eat to ensure peak well-being during the menopausal years.

Eating well

Here you will find the food and drink you need to eat before and during menopause to achieve specific health benefits. They are all so easy to incorporate into your daily meals that you will wonder why you – and your family – haven't tried them before.

The aim of getting your diet right is to help:

- control menopausal symptoms such as hot flashes, night sweats, vaginal dryness, lack of sex drive, lack of energy and mood swings
- prevent osteoporosis
- maintain a healthy heart
- protect against cancer
- minimize aching joints and stiffness
- prevent degenerative diseases like arthritis
- ensure good mental health
- slow the aging process
- control weight naturally – without dieting

Improving your health, which will enhance your quality of life, so you have sufficient energy for all your needs and develop a real zest for living.

Many of the foods recommended have several valuable qualities. Soy, for example, is perhaps best known for the phytoestrogens (plant hormones) it provides, but it also contains good levels of essential fatty acids, has antioxidant properties, is virtually free from saturated fats and has excellent levels of vegetable protein and a good fiber content. So eating one beneficial food can help your health in many different ways.

The essential ingredients

The following should all be included in your diet at menopause to optimize your health.

1. Phytoestrogens, including soy, lentils and chickpeas
2. Oily foods, including fish, nuts, seeds and oils
3. Plenty of fruit and vegetables
4. Complex carbohydrates, including oats, brown rice, whole grain bread
5. Plenty of fiber
6. Good fluid intake

1 Phytoestrogens

Since 1997, research into phytoestrogens – plant hormones – has exploded and they are now the subject of almost 4,000 medical papers a year. Phytoestrogens are not to be confused with xenoestrogens (see page 164), the gender-bending substances from plastics and pesticides that are causing so much havoc in the environment. On the contrary, phytoestrogens are thought to have a beneficial effect on health and are of special interest to women reaching menopause.

In clinical trials, phytoestrogens have been shown to reduce both hot flashes and night sweats.[1] One study published in *Obstetrics and Gynecology* showed that women taking soy capsules had a significant reduction in hot flashes in only four weeks compared to women who took dummy pills.[2] And phytoestrogens may have an even more crucial role in women's health, because studies are now taking place to see if they can help prevent breast cancer and heart disease.

The theory is that plant estrogens work in a special way and have a balancing effect on your hormones.[3] Eating soy, for example, can increase estrogen levels when they are low, but will not increase them unnecessarily (see page 10). That is why it can be helpful for reducing hot flashes at menopause (believed to be caused by a lack of estrogen) and still reduce the risk of breast cancer (often linked to an excess of estrogen).

THE JAPANESE EXPERIENCE

One of the questions that most perplexes scientists is why menopause is experienced so differently around the world. For example, up to 85 percent of

Western women will experience hot flashes[4] compared to only 14 percent in some Asian countries.[5]

Linked to this issue is the fact that in parts of the world, notably the Far East, breast cancer is not the major killer it is here in the West. Why? The UK seems to have a breast cancer death rate about six times higher than that in Japan, which gives us an important clue. Studies conducted in the U.S. have shown that when Japanese women move to the West, they are more likely to develop breast cancer[6]. Many experts think a major factor is diet, and this is borne out by the fact that as the traditional Japanese diet becomes more Westernized, the incidence of breast cancer in Japan is increasing.

There are a number of differences between the normal Japanese diet and ours. They eat a good quantity of unsaturated fats in oils and fish while the Western diet is high in saturated fat from meat and dairy foods. Traditionally, Japanese women do not eat much dairy food at all. The other main difference is their large consumption of soy bean products including tofu, miso (soy bean paste), tamari (wheat-free soy sauce), tempeh and soy milk. Many of these traditional soy foods are fermented, which makes them easier to digest. Fermented soy is found in soy sauce, tamari, miso, natto and tempeh, all different kinds of soy foods that are eaten in Japan. Tempeh is fermented in two days but miso and soy sauce can take many months.

The result is that the average Japanese woman's daily intake of isoflavones, the most beneficial phytoestrogen, is between 20 and 80 milligrams per day while American women generally consume between 1 and 3 milligrams per day. In fact, one recent study shows that healthy postmenopausal Caucasian women are consuming less than 1 milligram per day – quite a difference.[7]

WHY SOY HAS HAD A BAD PRESS

At the same time as all this good information about phytoestrogens has been emerging, there have also been negative statements, mostly about soy. Apart from concerns about genetic modification, for which soy is a prime candidate, there are claims that soy can accelerate brain aging, lead to thyroid disease and cause reproductive problems. Not surprisingly, women are confused. Many have written to me, perplexed about the findings and unsure whether they should be eating soy at all.

It is important to look at the source of the evidence. Many studies are funded by sponsors who can have a vested interest. If conflicting interests are involved you can find that positive studies being countered by negative ones.

Soy is now a major industry. It is used in margarines and salad dressings, to feed animals, and in newspaper printing ink. Many of the companies behind the research into soy accept and use the process of genetic modification. In other words, they produce GM foods. They fund research in the hope that studies will find that soy is completely safe or, even better, a wonder food we simply can't do without. But then the good publicity for soy tends to alarm another section of industry, the pharmaceutical giants who stand to lose a lot of money if alternatives to HRT and other menopausal drugs are found. The dairy industry, which would lose out if the population shifts to soy instead of milk and other diary products, is also affected. Everyone has something at stake. Who should you believe?

CAN SOY BE BAD FOR YOU?

Fortunately, there is little proof that soy can damage your health. In September 2000, the British Nutrition Foundation issued a statement saying: "Recent media coverage has raised a number of concerns about possible effects of soy products on health, including thyroid abnormalities, mineral deficiencies, Alzheimer's disease and effects in women consuming soy products during pregnancy on the unborn child.[8] In reality, for most of these there have been few published studies and much of the work cited to support many of these claims has been conducted in animals, rather than humans… These concerns remain speculative and unproven."

When you look closely at the research, it becomes obvious why it has produced such negative conclusions. In some of the studies mentioned in media scares, the animals were fed high amounts of raw soy flour for five years. In one study the scientists were looking at the effect of soy on the pancreas. The pancreas secretes trypsin, which enables your body to break down protein in the small intestine. Raw soy contains trypsin inhibitors that could theoretically stop this process from happening, causing an inflammation called pancreatitis. Even so, out of 26 monkeys tested, only one showed even moderate inflammation of the pancreas. The questions here are: Why use raw soy flour in tests and on animals? Who eats raw soy anyway?

The answer is that very few people do, either in the East, where soy is a traditional food source, or in the West where it is often used as a substitute for dairy foods. Traditionally fermented soy foods, such as Japanese miso and soy sauce, are relatively free of trypsin inhibitors. In tofu, these inhibitors end up in the soaking fluid (which is then discarded), not in the curd itself. Soy milk made from whole soy beans also involves a soaking process and again, the fluid is discarded.

A second point is that there is an enormous difference between whole soy beans and isolated compounds of soy. Most of the studies, and therefore the arguments, focus on isolated compounds. In other words, they are analyzing a part of the soy plant and not the whole food.

The soy used in clinical trials is usually soy protein isolate, made in an industrial setting. The fiber from the soy bean is removed with an alkaline solution and the beans are put into an aluminum tank with an acid wash. This is where concerns about Alzheimer's and aluminum come into play. You may remember an old cook's tip for cleaning out aluminum pans by cooking rhubarb in them to "wipe them clean." And it worked. The reason? The surface of the aluminum was neatly absorbed into the rhubarb. The same thing happens with soy beans. When left to soak in an aluminum tank, they absorb aluminum, which has been linked to dementia, because it has been found in patches of cell damage in the brains of people with Alzheimer's.

A very straightforward concept, and certainly relevant to soy protein isolates, but not whole soy foods. Furthermore, soy protein isolates undergo a number of other chemical treatments that add nitrates to the end product. Nitrates are another concern, as they are known to be implicated in cancer.

So it seems the problem lies not with foods made from whole soy but with the soy protein isolates frequently used in convenience foods. These turn up in textured vegetable protein (often with added "chicken" or "beef" flavoring), hydrolyzed vegetable protein (used as flavor enhancers in soups and sauces), lecithin (which thickens products such as mayonnaise), and even infant formulas, children's snacks and some soy milks. Up to 60 percent of processed foods contain soy, including bread, biscuits, pizza and baby food and in the majority of cases, the soy takes the form of powdered soy isolate, and is not derived from whole soy beans. But this is not the kind of soy that Japanese women benefit from.

In addition to the fact that soy isolate has infiltrated a good part of our food supply, there is concern that some is genetically modified. This is important because genetically modified soy contains fewer phytoestrogens than the non-genetically modified variety.[9]

The only way you can tell exactly what soy a product contains is to read the label. Some manufacturers buy soy isolate powder and make it into soy milk by adding other ingredients. Other companies specify on the label that their products are made from whole beans, and they also confirm that these beans are not genetically modified.

The thyroid and soy connection

Some foods are termed "goitrogens," which means that they have the ability to block the uptake of iodine from the blood. Iodine is essential for thyroid function, and a deficiency can be the cause of an underactive thyroid condition. Therefore, any food that is a goitrogen will make an underactive thyroid problem worse. Soy is one of those foods, but so are turnips, cabbage, peanuts, pine nuts, Brussels sprouts, broccoli, kale and millet, when eaten raw. If you are diagnosed with a severe underactive thyroid, you will normally be told to restrict your intake of these foods. When eaten raw, and in excess, problems can occur.

This does not mean that people with an underactive thyroid should never eat soy, just that they should be careful to limit their intake. There is an abounding myth that if a little of something is good for you, a lot must be even better. I often see this belief illustrated in nutrition, where people tend to believe that taking extra quantities of herbs or vitamin supplements will enhance the effect. Very often the effects of a food or supplement are most beneficial at a specific, often small dose.

The same applies to soy. News of its benefits has led to a boom in soy products and it is now available in almost every imaginable form. In fact, you can buy snack bars that are nothing more than raw, ground soy beans. Remember the problem with the monkeys and raw soy flour? The same goes here. Soy is not meant to be eaten raw, or in excessive quantities.

Mineral absorption

The final criticism of soy is that it can interfere with the absorption of minerals. To a certain extent this is true, although as we shall see, that may not be a bad thing. Soy beans are certainly high in phytates, which can block the uptake of essential minerals such as calcium, magnesium, iron and zinc. But the action of these phytates may be one of the reasons why soy seems to have a protective effect against cancer. This is because the phytates in the soy act as antioxidants, controlling the action of substances like iron that can generate the free radicals known to cause cancer or heart disease (see page 171).

Phytates are not only found in soy beans. They are present in the bran or husks of all grains and legumes.

EAT PHYTOESTROGENS!

So eat soy products – they are good for you! But eat them in their traditional form, choosing products such as miso, tofu, or organic soy milk. These foods are healthy and can have a dramatic effect on your health, particularly during menopause. Avoid gimmicky soy bars and snacks unless you know they are made from the whole bean and even then, make sure that the beans are not raw or genetically modified.

Variety is the key to a healthy diet, and it's important to remember that soy is only one of many phytoestrogens (see page 135). My suggestion is to incorporate a selection of different phytoestrogens in your diet. If you want to make life easy, concentrate on beans because the isoflavones they contain seem to be the most beneficial type of phytoestrogen at menopause. Beans are easy to use and are very tasty when added to salads, soups and casseroles. Most beans (except for lentils) need to be soaked, sometimes overnight, before cooking. Alternatively, you can buy organic beans in cans from most supermarkets. For details of the use of soy or isoflavone supplements for menopause, see page 135 of this book.

Where to find phytoestrogens

The following are rich sources of phytoestrogens:

• legumes including soy, lentils, chickpeas, aduki beans, kidney beans, peas
• garlic
• celery
• seeds, including flax seed, sesame, pumpkin, poppy, caraway, sunflower
• grains, such as rice, oats, wheat, barley, rye
• fruit, including apples, plums, cherries
• vegetables, including broccoli, carrots, rhubarb, potatoes
• sprouts, such as alfalfa and mung bean sprouts
• some herbs and spices such as cinnamon, sage, red clover, hops, fennel and parsley

2 Oils

It may come as a surprise to discover that oily foods such as fish, nuts, and seeds are good for you. For years, anything associated with fat or oil has been rejected by thousands of women following low-fat and no-fat diets. Such women frequently complain of symptoms such as dry skin, lifeless hair, cracked nails, fatigue, depression, dry eyes, lack of motivation, aching joints,

Phytoestrogens explained

Not all phytoestrogens are the same – there are many different types. The most relevant are:

• Isoflavones, found in legumes such as soy, lentils and chickpeas. These are the most beneficial class of phytoestrogen. They can be broken down into four other types: genistein, daidzein, biochanin A and formononentin. Chickpeas and lentils contain all four, while soy contains just genistein and daidzein. All are inactive until converted by bacteria in the gut into substances that have an estrogenic action.
• Lignans form part of most cereals and vegetables, with the highest concentrations in seeds that give oils, especially flax seed.
• Coumestans are found mainly in alfalfa and mung bean sprouts.

forgetfulness, breast pain and even difficulty in losing weight – all symptoms that could be "blamed" on menopause. But they can equally be signs of an essential fatty acid (EFA) deficiency.

It is because these fats are essential to your health that they are known as "essential fatty acids" while others are not. Essential fats "oil" the body by lubricating the joints, skin and vagina and are a vital component of every human cell. They help to balance hormones, insulate nerve cells, keep skin and arteries supple and the body warm. In addition, they can boost your metabolism and even help with weight loss. Your body also makes beneficial prostaglandins (hormone-like substances) from these essential fatty acids, so they are particularly useful at menopause. Because they help to lower blood pressure, decrease inflammation and lower sodium levels, they can ease problems such as painful joints and water retention.

As the body cannot make essential fats, your only source is food. If your diet is too low in EFAs, serious problems such as heart disease, cancer, arthritis and depression can result. Unfortunately, all too often such illnesses are viewed as part of the degenerative process of getting older – "just one of those things."

EFAs are found in nuts, seeds, oily fish and vegetables and you should try to make these a regular part of your diet. A handful of nuts or a salad dressing made with good quality oil can be sufficient intake each day.

One particularly good source of EFAs is flax oil (linseed oil). This can be highly beneficial at menopause because it contains both types of essential fatty acid. It not only supplies the Omega 6 oils found in other seeds but also provides a quantity of Omega 3 oil as well. In fact, the Latin name for flax seed is *Linum usitatissimum*, the second part of which means "most useful" – which indeed it is.

Flax seed are also rich in phytoestrogens called lignans, which are anti-viral, anti-fungal and antibacterial and have a beneficial estrogenic action. A regular intake of lignans has been associated with lower incidence of cancer of the breast, ovaries, uterus and colon, and prostate in men.[10]

To increase the absorption of the nutrients from flax seed, put them in a grinder or lightly crack them before sprinkling them on your food. For a good balance of essential fatty acids, combine the flax seed with sesame, sunflower and pumpkin seeds, which also have excellent antioxidant properties (see below).

Oily fish, such as mackerel, sardines, tuna, herrings and salmon, are another rich source of essential fats. A small portion of salmon (4 ounces) can contain up to 3,600 milligrams of Omega 3 fatty acids while the same size piece of cod accounts for only 300 milligrams. A small piece of oily fish can supply almost half your protein requirements for a day as well as providing good levels of B12 and iodine, essential for healthy thyroid gland function and an efficient metabolism.

Despite the concerns about the pollutants that are in the sea and therefore also in the fish, it is important to eat some fish at least two to three times a week.

BOTTLED OILS

You can top up your consumption of the natural oils found in nuts, seeds and fish with bottled oils, used for salad dressings and cooking. What you may not realize is that careful choice, storage and use of oils is vital as they can be easily damaged, resulting in negative effects on your health.

Where to find essential fats

- Extra virgin olive oil for cooking and also salad dressings, combined with other oils such as flax seed
- Nuts (almonds, pecan, brazil and so on) and seeds (sesame, pumpkin, sunflower, etc.)
- Nut butters made without sugar or palm oil
- Tahini (creamed sesame seeds) for sauces and dressings
- Oily fish such as mackerel, sardines, herring, salmon and tuna

---

Antioxidants and free radicals

Antioxidants are perhaps the most important nutrients of all because they protect against the effects of free radicals. You might wonder why you need antioxidants when oxygen is the basis of all plant and animal life and is vital for survival. But paradoxically, it can also be highly dangerous.

The normal biochemical reactions that take place in your body make oxygen unstable, resulting in the "oxidation" of other molecules. These generate harmful substances called free radicals, which are also triggered by pollution, smoking, fried or barbecued food and UV rays from the sun. These highly reactive chemical fragments speed up the aging process and susceptibility to disease by destroying healthy cells. They also attack collagen, the "cement" that holds cells together, which is the primary constituent of bone, cartilage and connective tissue. As you get older there is a decrease in collagen, which can cause changes to your skin (wrinkles, prominent veins, slow wound healing, bruising easily) nails (brittleness), eyes (dryness, dark circles under the eyes), gums (bleeding, infections), hair (dullness, split ends, poor growth, hair loss) and mouth (bad breath, mouth ulcers). Not an attractive prospect. Free radicals can also attack the DNA in the nucleus of a cell, causing cell mutation, which is why they have been linked to cancer, coronary heart disease and rheumatoid arthritis. So it is very important to protect yourself from the cell damage caused by free radicals with foods that are rich in antioxidants.

Where to find antioxidants

Vitamin A	Orange and yellow fruits and vegetables (mangos, carrots, pumpkins); oily fish
Vitamin C	Fruits (particularly citrus); green leafy vegetables such as broccoli; cauliflower; berries; potatoes and sweet potatoes
Vitamin E	Nuts and seeds; avocados; vegetable oils; oily fish
Selenium	Brazil nuts; tuna; cabbage
Zinc	Pumpkin and sunflower seeds; fish; almonds

If an oil is overheated, left in sunlight, or reused after cooking, oxidation may take place. This leaves the oil open to attack by free radicals. To restrict free radical formation, choose cold-pressed unrefined vegetable oils or extra-virgin olive oil. Unfortunately most standard supermarket oils (but not the cold-pressed or extra virgin oils) are processed using chemicals and heat to obtain the maximum amount of oil from each batch, and anti-foaming agents may also be added. Both destroy the quality and nutritional content of the oil. The best advice is to choose organic oils, available from health food stores and a number of supermarkets. Store the oil away from sunlight as light can damage the quality.

It is equally important to take care with oils used for cooking, especially when frying. Choose olive oil or butter for this because they are less likely to cause free radicals than polyunsaturated fats such as sunflower oil, which become unstable when heated. Reduce the temperature to minimize the chances of free radicals forming and try to bake, steam, roast or grill instead. And still use olive oil even when baking or roasting.

3 Fruit and vegetables

Eating plenty of fruit and vegetables is important for a number of reasons. They contain a good supply of vitamins and minerals, including vital antioxidants, and

---

Fats: essential, good, and bad

The type of fat you eat can make the world of difference to your health so it is important to learn to distinguish between them, not simply to cut fat out altogether.

Polyunsaturated fats are vital for your health. They can be split into two types:

• Omega 6 help to prevent blood clots and keep the blood thin. They can also reduce inflammation and pain in the joints and so are vital to prevent arthritis. Good sources are nuts (such as walnuts) and seeds (such as sunflower) plus soy and flax seed, which are rich in phytoestrogens (see page 54). Omega 6 EFAs are also found in evening primrose, starflower and borage oil.
• Omega 3 can mop up harmful free radicals that cause cell damage. They help to lower blood pressure, reduce the risk of heart disease, soften the skin, increase immune function, increase metabolic rate, improve energy levels and alleviate eczema. They are found in oily fish and are also present to some extent in flax seed, pumpkin seeds, walnuts and dark green vegetables.

continued

> Monounsaturated fats, also known as Omega 9 fats, are thought to lower LDL ("bad") cholesterol and raise HDL ("good") cholesterol. The high consumption of olive oil, high in monounsaturated fats, is thought to be one of the factors that contribute to the low rate of heart disease in Mediterranean countries.
>
> Saturated fats (see page 172) should not form a large part of your diet because they can lead to the production of "bad" prostaglandins that can cause joint swelling and pain.

fiber to help your body adjust to menopause. In order to benefit fully from the health-giving properties of fruit and vegetables, you need to eat a wide variety (preferably organic). Eating five pieces a day will help you to absorb a plentiful supply of vitamins C, E and beta-carotene (the plant form of vitamin A), all of which have antioxidant properties, as do the minerals selenium and zinc.

Some important plant chemicals (phytochemicals) are also powerful antioxidants. They include lycopene (found in tomatoes), bioflavonoids (in citrus fruits) and proanthocyanidins (in berries, grapes and green tea). You can find more information on these in my *Eat Your Way Through the Menopause* cookbook.

If you cannot buy fresh vegetables, frozen are better than canned. Dried fruit – raisins, apricots, dates, currants, prunes, figs, apple rings and so on – can also be eaten in moderation provided that you read the label and avoid any that contain the preserving agent sulphur dioxide, also used as a bleaching agent in flour. Sulphur dioxide occurs naturally and is produced chemically for commercial use, but it is suspected of being a factor in genetic mutations and can also irritate the digestive tract. It is often used as a color enhancer and is frequently added to dried apricots to keep them orange. Fruits that are free from preservatives often turn brown (which is why figs and dates are usually free from sulphur dioxide) but taste fine.

Another additive to avoid is mineral oil. This is often applied to dried fruits such as mixed fruit, raisins and currants because it gives them a shiny appearance and keeps them separate. Unfortunately mineral oil can interfere with the absorption of calcium. As it passes through your body, it can pick up and excrete the oil-soluble vitamins A, D, E and K that you really want to retain.

4 Complex carbohydrates

Carbohydrates give you energy and help to increase serotonin levels, the "calming" brain chemical that helps to lift mood and curb appetite. The

Why choose organic?

Organic produce usually contains more of the most valuable nutrients than non-organic food. This is because one of the practices of organic farming involves crop rotation, which ensures that the soil is enriched rather than depleted.

Fruit and vegetables
Because organic produce is grown without pesticides, organic vegetables such as carrots and potatoes do not need to be peeled. This is an advantage because most of the nutrients of vegetables and fruits are concentrated just under the skin. Just scrub them carefully, with water, and prepare as normal.

Grains
If your budget is limited and you are unsure of what to prioritize, go for organic grains. Grains are very small and can absorb more pesticides than other foods, so even if this is the only organic part of your diet, it can make a huge difference.

Dairy
Choose organic brands to avoid the harmful effects of antibiotics and other chemicals that may have been added to the animals' feed. Of all the dairy foods, yogurt is the most beneficial for your health, but only when it contains beneficial bacteria that are found naturally in the digestive system. (Look for the words "live" or "bio" on the carton.) These friendly bacteria defend the immune system and help to keep unhealthy bacteria, fungal infections and viruses at bay. When yogurt is heat-treated it loses its original culture.

Eggs
Organic free-range eggs are the ones to choose. Free-range is certainly kinder to animals but the birds can still be fed an inappropriate diet, which can include chemicals and antibiotics. Organic hens have a strict dietary regime, without worrying additives.

amount of energy they provide depends on the form in which you eat them. Carbohydrates are starches and sugars, and can either be "simple" or "complex." The more complex the carbohydrate, the greater the health benefits. Complex carbohydrates give you sustained energy (stopping you feeling tired), balance your blood sugar (so minimizing cravings and stabilizing your appetite), lower cholesterol and greatly reduce menopausal symptoms.

With the exception of fruit, most simple carbohydrates are refined foods from which the goodness has been stripped away. It is important to ensure that your carbohydrates are unrefined if you are to obtain the benefits associated with complex carbohydrates. In general terms, this means choosing "whole" and "brown," instead of "white." Whole wheat bread, brown rice and whole grain flour are rich in essential vitamins, minerals, trace elements and valuable fiber, while their refined counterparts have been stripped of these. Some manufacturers now "replace" lost nutrients by adding vitamins and minerals to the final product, but these are still nutritionally inferior to the whole versions. A particular problem is that they lack fiber, essential to slow the digestive process and release a steady flow of energy.

WHERE TO FIND CARBOHYDRATES

Complex carbohydrates
- Grains (wheat, rye, oats, rice, barley, corn)
- Beans (lentils, kidney beans, soy, etc.)
- Vegetables

Simple carbohydrates
- Honey
- Sugar
- Fruit

5 Natural fiber

Fiber is well known for its action on the bowel, but it has a number of other health benefits too. Most people are aware that fiber increases the bulk of stools so that they are easier to eliminate from the body, thus preventing constipation. It does this by binding with water – so it is important to make sure your fluid intake is adequate if you increase the amount of fiber in your diet. By encouraging regular bowel action, fiber stops the putrefaction and fermentation that take place when food stays in the bowel too long, which can lead to problems of bloating and flatulence that are particularly common during menopause. Fiber also helps to prevent disease. It can ward off bowel conditions such as colon cancer, lower cholesterol levels, neutralize harmful toxins and balance hormones.

Less well known is fiber's role in slowing the absorption of sugars and maintaining blood sugar balance (see page 67). Without fiber, food acts more quickly on your levels of blood sugar and is harder to eliminate from the body.

The bulkiness of fiber also helps you feel full after meals. This encourages you to feel more satisfied with what you have eaten and reduces any tendency to overeat.

There are two main types of fiber, insoluble (found in whole grains and vegetables) and soluble (found in grains such as oats and rice, fruit and beans). Soluble fiber is especially important to women because it locks onto estrogen so that it is excreted more efficiently. Soluble fiber stops "old" estrogens passed out via the bile from entering the bloodstream again, preventing any excess build-up of estrogen. As the problems associated with excess estrogen include breast cancer, fibroids and endometriosis, it is especially important to eat enough soluble fiber if you take HRT, to ensure that you eliminate the estrogen efficiently and prevent it from recirculating.

Although there has been a great deal of interest in fiber in recent years, the focus has often been on adding bran to food to increase the fiber content. However, this misses the point. Despite its associations with whole foods, bran is a refined food that has been stripped from the grains of cereal plants. Bran also contains phytates that have a binding effect on vital nutrients such as iron, zinc and magnesium, making these minerals less easy to absorb. What is more, phytates also bind to calcium, making it harder for the body to absorb a mineral that is essential for bone health, especially during menopause. Eating so much "roughage" can also lead to gastrointestinal problems and aggravate conditions such as irritable bowel syndrome. It can actually make bloating worse.

WHERE TO FIND NATURAL FIBER
• Fresh fruit and vegetables (cooked and raw)
• Whole grains such as brown rice, oats, whole grain bread, nuts, beans and seeds.

6 Fluids

You can survive without food for about five weeks but you will only last five days without fluids. Your body is made up of approximately 70 percent water, which is essential for every function of the body, from absorption and digestion to circulation and excretion. You need water to carry nutrients into cells, remove waste, and also to maintain body temperature, which is important for women suffering from hot flashes and night sweats.

Most people do not drink enough water and ironically women who suffer from water retention often drink less than most. They restrict their liquid intake thinking that the less they drink, the less their bodies will retain. Actually, the opposite is true. If you restrict how much you drink, your body tries to compensate and will retain liquid, thinking that it is in short supply.

Ideally, you should try to drink around six glasses of water a day, in place of other less healthy drinks. An excellent start to the day is a cup of hot water and a slice of lemon, which is wonderfully refreshing and excellent for the liver. Herbal teas can be counted as part of your liquid intake but drinks such as coffee, black tea and alcohol should not as they act as diuretics.

Unfortunately, tap water may be contaminated with any number of impurities, which vary from area to area. Arsenic, lead and copper can all occur naturally in tap water and even if the water is pure to start with, it can be contaminated by the pipes that transport it. Other substances such as pesticides and fertilizers can leach into water through the ground.

Although filtering drinking water won't eliminate every impurity, it will help to remove a variety of contaminants, including, in some cases, xenoestrogens (see page 152). You can buy a jug filter or have one installed under the sink. The second option makes it easier to use filtered water for washing fruit and vegetables as well as for cooking and drinking.

Water sources

Whichever type of bottled water you prefer, try to buy it in glass bottles rather than plastic, which can contaminate the water with xenoestrogens. Here is a guide to what's what.

• Spring water is taken from one or more underground sources and may undergo a range of treatments, such as filtration and blending.
• Natural mineral water is bottled straight from the source and is not treated in any way. The supply has to be officially registered, and conform to purity standards, and carry details of its source and mineral analysis on the bottle.
• Naturally sparkling water is water taken from its underground source with enough natural carbon dioxide to make it bubbly.
• Carbonated water has carbon dioxide added during bottling, in the same way as ordinary fizzy drinks.

CHAPTER 6

What Not to Eat at Menopause

There is a lot you can do to minimize menopausal symptoms and improve your health by introducing new foods into your diet. But there are also elements in the diet that could actually make menopause more troublesome and increase your chances of getting osteoporosis or heart problems.

It is no good planning healthy meals that incorporate phytoestrogens, antioxidants and essential fatty acids, for example, if at the same time you are eating foods that disrupt your hormones, leach calcium from your bones and are detrimental to your general health. You will simply be fighting a losing battle.

That doesn't mean that you have to give up your favorite indulgences. There are only a few foods you need to reduce or eliminate, and there's no need to be too rigid about it. If you eat fairly well at home, the occasional slip on a vacation or when you are invited out to dinner will not make too much difference. Just make sure that the foundation of your diet is good.

The importance of blood sugar

Have a look at this list of symptoms: mood swings, irritability, aggressive outbursts, crying spells, anxiety, tension, excessive sweating, depression, tiredness, forgetfulness and lack of concentration.

As you can see, they look exactly like symptoms of menopause, but the truth is that all these symptoms can also be due to fluctuations in blood sugar. It is very common for a woman of 45-plus to be told that she is menopausal and needs HRT when she says she has these symptoms, even if she still has regular periods. It is too easy to blame every health problem that women experience in mid-life on menopause, and they all need to be checked out. After all, a number of women have told me that their male partners get night sweats too, and those definitely aren't due to menopause!

THE STRESS CONNECTION

If your blood sugar (glucose) level drops, your body automatically releases adrenaline – a major stress hormone – into the bloodstream to prompt your liver to produce more glucose to counteract the fall. It is this release of adrenaline that produces symptoms that mimic menopause.

If your blood sugar levels often dip during the day, adrenaline will be pumped around your body on a regular basis. This can take a toll on your health, especially at menopause. The body experiences all the sensations listed above even though there is no outside stress to respond to.

Another unwanted consequence of rollercoaster blood sugar levels is the wear and tear on the adrenal glands. These were never intended to pump out adrenaline regularly during the day and repeated stimulation can interfere with their functioning. The results can be particularly disturbing during menopause because the adrenal glands produce the hormone estrone, which takes over as the main source of estrogen when your ovaries stop production. If your adrenal glands are under pressure, they will be not be able to supply this estrogen and you may start to get symptoms such as feeling tired all the time, weight gain, mood swings and food cravings. So it is crucial that your adrenal glands are in the best possible condition and do not become exhausted through overwork.

Luckily it is relatively easy to tell whether your symptoms are produced by stress or menopause. Because fluctuations in blood sugar are governed by how and what you eat, you can make changes and see what happens to your symptoms. If they disappear, they were caused by a drop in your blood sugar and were not menopausal.

It also helps to analyze your symptoms. When women tell me they get night sweats, I ask, "Does the night sweat wake you up or do you wake up and start sweating a split second later?" If you wake and then get a sweat, it is usually caused by a drop in blood sugar during the night, rather than by menopause. When blood sugar reaches a low point – usually at around 3 to 4 o'clock in the morning – adrenaline kicks in and wakes you up, which is followed by sweating.

Low blood sugar can interrupt sleep in other ways too. A common experience is when a woman falls asleep as soon as her head hits the pillow but wakes up suddenly in the middle of the night, her heart racing. Waking up with a start and palpitations can be caused by adrenaline surging through the body as the blood sugar drops. During the day, on the other hand, the degree to which your blood sugar levels rise and fall depends on two main factors – what you eat and drink and when you eat and drink.

WHAT SHOULD HAPPEN

When your body is in balance, it regulates its own blood sugar levels without any sudden highs or lows. During digestion, glucose (sugar) is drawn through the wall of the intestine into the bloodstream. At this point, your blood sugar level is naturally quite high. Your body takes what it needs for energy and then produces insulin from the pancreas to lower the level. The remaining glucose is changed into glycogen and stored in the liver and muscles, to be used later, and blood sugar levels return to normal.

To maintain a steady blood sugar level during the day, you need foods that give a slow rise in blood sugar and maintain that level for about three hours. You should then have something to eat before it drops, but sweet snacks are not the answer. What you need are complex carbohydrates (rye, oats, rice) that give a slow release of energy because it takes time for the digestive tract to break them down. Aim to eat complex carbohydrates as part of your main meals together with protein, and you will find that this small change can make an enormous difference to the way you feel throughout the day.

As we've seen, if you wake during the night – at around 3 or 4 o'clock – and cannot get back to sleep, it is likely that your blood sugar level has dropped and adrenaline has kicked in. Eating a small, starchy snack, such as half a slice of rye bread or a rice cake, one hour before going to bed will help you to sleep through the night.

THE BLOOD SUGAR ROLLERCOASTER

UP ...

Some foods give your blood sugar levels an instant but short-lived boost followed by an equally sharp fall. Refined foods, such as sugar and white flour, are no longer in their "whole" state, and have been stripped of their natural goodness by various manufacturing processes. As a result, they are digested very quickly and glucose enters the bloodstream rapidly. In addition, your body has to use its supply of vitamins and minerals to digest refined foods, so depleting your own stores. Stimulants such as tea, coffee, alcohol and chocolate also affect your blood sugar, causing a sharp and fast rise in blood glucose followed by a rapid drop. At this low point, you will feel tired and drained and need something like a bar of chocolate or cup of coffee (or both!) to give you a boost. This boost makes the blood sugar level soar and the cycle is repeated. You are back on the rollercoaster ride of blood sugar highs and lows.

If your blood sugar level rises too high, insulin is produced to lower it, a condition called hyperglycemia. If the body cannot produce enough insulin to deal with the glucose, diabetes may result and insulin supplements will be needed to control the blood sugar level.

... AND DOWN

Blood sugar that stays low for a period of time (hypoglycemia) can cause symptoms that are virtually identical to menopausal ones. If there is a long gap since you last ate (over three hours for women), your blood sugar will drop to quite a low level. You feel the need for a quick boost (a cup of tea or a cookie). Many women experience this around 3 or 4 o'clock in the afternoon when they hit a slump and feel they need something to keep them going. But the consequence of succumbing to a sugar rush is that adrenaline is released from the adrenal glands and glucagon, which works in the opposite way to insulin, is produced from the pancreas. Glucagon increases blood glucose by encouraging the liver to turn some of its glycogen stores into glucose. The result is a high blood sugar level that calls on the pancreas to over-produce insulin in order to reduce glucose levels. The rollercoaster starts all over again and the adrenal glands (and you!) become more exhausted.

The stress hormone

Adrenaline is known as the "fight or flight" hormone and its effect is very powerful. It is meant to be released in times of danger, when your body senses a mental or physical threat. It provokes the following immediate and dramatic response:

• The liver releases stored sugar into the bloodstream to give you energy for "fight or flight."
• Blood is diverted from the skin into muscles and internal organs. Your heart speeds up and the arteries constrict to raise your blood pressure, sending blood to where it is needed most.
• Your blood thickens, ready to clot, in case you are injured.
• Your digestion shuts down because all energy is diverted to the organs that need it most. This all means that you are prepared to run faster, fight back and react more quickly than normal.

How to balance your blood sugar

Avoid:
• refined carbohydrates, and "white" in general. Remember that white flour is in many things such as cakes, cookies, pastries and white bread.
• sugar or the foods it is in, including chocolate, sweets, cookies, pastries and soft drinks
• tea, coffee (also decaffeinated), alcohol
• soft drinks
• convenience foods, as they are likely to contain refined carbohydrates
• smoking

but include instead:
• unrefined complex carbohydrates, including whole wheat bread, brown rice, millet, oats, rye, etc.
• good-quality protein such as fish, eggs, nuts, seeds, beans
• fruits and diluted pure fruit juice
• breakfast – it's essential. Oat products such as oatmeal are good choices.
• small, frequent meals no more than three hours apart.
• herbal teas, grain coffees, fruit teas

Foods that can harm

1 Sugar

When sugar is in its natural form – whole sugar cane – it is fine to eat, as it is a whole food. The problem starts when it is refined. Processing removes the fiber as well as the vitamins, minerals and trace elements, leaving pure sugar, which is easily eaten in excess. And we do. On average, each of us consumes 2.25 pounds of sugar per week, and much of this is "invisible" sugar, hidden in different, and not necessarily sweet, foods. In 1850, the world production of sugar was 1.5 million tons per year; that has now risen 75 million tons. We are eating 25 times the amount of sugar we ate 200 years ago.[1]

Refined sugar is just empty calories and provides no nutritional value. In fact, its effect on your metabolism makes it more difficult for you to lose weight. Every time you eat, your body has a choice: it can burn that food as energy or it can store it as fat. Scientists know that if more insulin is released, more of your food is converted into fat. What's more, the process of converting food into fat protects your fat stores and prevents existing fat from being broken down. So the more sugar you eat, the more insulin your body releases, and the more fat it stores.

It has also been found that sugar detrimentally affects the ability of the disease-fighting white blood cells to engulf and consume bacteria and foreign substances.[2] So sugar can also damage your immune system and compromise your body's ability to fight infection.

Because of the harm it can do to your health and the negative effects it has on menopausal symptoms, I suggest that you eliminate sugar completely. If you routinely add it to drinks such as tea or foods like fruit or cereals, try to wean yourself off it, and avoid eating obviously sweet foods, such as chocolate. Hidden sugar is another problem to watch out for, and it is found in the most unlikely places. Sugar is added to a wide range of foods, from canned vegetables and soups to yogurt and even pasta sauces, because it is an inexpensive bulking agent. It is important to read the labels. A fruit yogurt, for example, can contain up to eight teaspoons of sugar and a "healthy" granola bar can have the same. You may be surprised to hear that even toothpaste can contain sugar. As toothpaste is not a food, the sugar doesn't have to be listed as an ingredient.

Be wary of food labels that say "no added sugar." It can mean either no added sugar of any kind (good) or simply no added sucrose (not so good). Don't assume that sugar content is very low because the packet bears a "no added sugar" label. In order to make the sugar content look less, the manufacturers break down the sugars into various forms, although they all have relatively the same effect on your body. Any words ending in "-ose" are sugars, so when reading labels compare the total sugar figures provided. Look out for:

- Fructose – fruit sugar
- Glucose – blood sugar found in the body, fast-acting
- Dextrose – sugar from cornstarch, chemically identical to glucose
- Lactose – milk sugar
- Maltose – made from starch
- Sucrose – common table sugar, made from sugar cane or beets

If you are tempted to substitute artificial sweeteners for sugar (see page 69), don't. You are simply introducing an alien chemical into the body and giving it extra work to do. Although it may be hard at first, as you give up sugar, your taste buds will adapt. The natural sweetness of foods, such as parsnips and sweet potatoes, will become evident and much more attractive while sweetened, processed foods will begin to taste overly sweet. If you do find you need a sweetener for some foods, try small amounts of honey, maple syrup, brown rice syrup and barley malt syrup. These are healthier alternatives because (unlike sugar) they have some nutritional value, and are also less likely to cause huge swings in your blood sugar levels.

Make an exception for fruit

Although it is important to avoid sugars where possible, there is one exception – fruit. Fruit contains fructose (fruit sugar) but it is also a good source of fiber, which slows digestion. Stick to whole fruit rather than pure fruit juice, which can cause a rapid change in blood sugar levels because it is not buffered by fiber. You absorb a much higher level of fructose by drinking fruit juice than by eating a piece of fruit. One glass of orange juice can contain the same amount of fructose as eight oranges, but while you could drink the juice in a few moments, you would be most unlikely to eat eight oranges at one sitting. If you want to drink fruit juice, dilute it to make it less concentrated.

---

2 Artificial sweeteners

If a food or drink is described as being "low sugar," "diet" or "low calorie," it usually contains a chemical sweetener such as aspartame. Artificial sweeteners can also be found in some popsicles, sauces, instant noodles and even medicines (check the labels carefully).

Women are often misled into believing that artificial sweeteners help to control weight. Ironically, however, it has been found that people who regularly use artificial sweeteners tend to gain weight because these sweeteners increase the appetite.[3] Aspartame is 180 times sweeter than sugar and it can lead to binge-eating and weight problems.

Aspartame has also been linked to mood swings and depression because it alters the levels of the brain chemical serotonin.[4] It works in exactly the opposite way to SSRIs (Selective Serotonin Reuptake Inhibitors), one of the classes of drug used for depression designed to maximize serotonin, which helps to lift mood and reduce appetite. Given that volatile moods and depression are two of the prime emotional symptoms linked with menopause, it makes sense to avoid aspartame and any foods or drinks that contain it.

Besides worries about its effect on mood and weight, there are other concerns about aspartame. The Aspartame Toxicity Information Center (www.holisticmed.com/aspartame) has been set up in response to fears that the sweetener may be causing serious health problems. In addition to psychological problems such as low mood, depression and memory loss, there are a variety of physical symptoms linked to regular consumption of aspartame, from numbness and tingling to skin problems such as urticaria and rashes, seizures and convulsions, headaches, eye problems and nausea and vomiting.

Aspartame releases three substances during digestion that can have an adverse effect on your health. The first is methanol, which converts to formaldehyde (a toxin in the same group as cyanide and arsenic) and formic acid.[5] The others are two amino acids, aspartic acid and phenylalanine. Amino acids are fundamental constituents of all proteins, but they are normally ingested in small quantities and in combination with other amino aids. In this case, however, aspartic acid and phenylalanine are produced in isolation and in much larger quantities than usual, affecting the way the brain uses amino acids.[6] There is also a suspicion that aspartame is addictive, and that people who drink a large number (three to four cans) of diet soft drinks every day, or regularly chew sugar-free gum, may experience withdrawal symptoms if they stop.

My advice is to avoid any foods or drinks that contain artificial sweeteners. You will need to read the labels as they can be found in everything from fizzy drinks to yogurt, desserts, canned foods, many convenience foods and much, much more.

3 Stimulants

Stimulants such as sugar, caffeine (in tea, coffee and chocolate) and alcohol trigger a sugar rush in your blood followed by a drop that contributes to the rollercoaster rise and fall of blood sugar levels. Stimulants can increase hot flashes by making the blood vessels dilate. Just hot drinks themselves can worsen hot flashes. Indeed, you may have noticed the connection between drinking a cup of tea or coffee and the start of a hot flash. When you drink something hot on a summer's day, it helps you to cool down by dilating the blood vessels and encouraging sweating. The same is true of spicy foods such as curries, so keep these to a minimum during menopause if they kick-start a hot flash for you.

A wider problem with alcohol, tea and coffee is that they are "social poisons," acceptable drugs that have an anti-depressant or stimulant effect. Because they are so widely used, it is easy to forget about their addictive side. However, during menopause it is especially important to look at their effects on your health and ask if the pleasure is worth the price. When you are young, you are able to eliminate toxins more easily and have the resilience to burn the candle at both ends. But as you grow older, the effects accumulate and your body becomes less tolerant, as if to say, "If you keep putting this junk in me, I will just get slower, sicker, and look and feel older than my years."

Caffeine

A cup of instant coffee contains around 66 milligrams of caffeine and filtered coffee contains even more. Even tea contains around 50 milligrams per cup. Caffeine is a diuretic that can flush vital nutrients and trace elements out of the body. The active ingredients in caffeine called methylxanthines are found in coffee (even decaffeinated), chocolate, cola drinks, cocoa, tea (black and green) and some medications containing caffeine, such as painkillers. These have been linked to a benign breast condition known as fibrocystic disease and to breast pain, or mastalgia. Many women experience breast discomfort the week before their period and this can become worse, and occur at any time of month, as you reach your 40s. Simply cutting out caffeine can help to bring relief from painful, tender breasts.

Tannin

The tannin in tea binds important minerals and prevents the body from absorbing them. During menopause, when you need to maximize your intake of calcium, zinc, iron and magnesium, it is essential to do everything you can to help your body make use of these important minerals. Otherwise, you could find that although you are eating a nutritious diet and perhaps even taking vitamin and mineral supplements, these vital nutrients are wasted because they are excreted rather than absorbed.

If you don't want to give up tea entirely, drink green tea (*Camellia sinensis*). Green tea comes from the same plant as ordinary black tea but its leaves are not fermented. Although it contains a small amount of caffeine, it also contains polyphenols (antioxidants) which have been credited with a range of health benefits.

Alcohol

Alcohol is made by the action of yeast on sugar, so it is full of calories. One glass of wine supplies about 100 calories and a pint of beer around 200 calories.

Alcohol can contribute to blood sugar swings and acts as an "anti-nutrient," depleting the body of vitamins and minerals, especially zinc. Alcohol also interferes with the metabolism of essential fatty acids needed to produce prostaglandins, the chemicals that help to control vascular reactions such as hot flashes. Most important of all, alcohol compromises the function of the liver.

It is important to keep your liver healthy at menopause as it is the waste-disposal unit of the body, ridding it of toxins such as waste products, drugs and alcohol, and also unwanted hormones. If your liver is not functioning efficiently, old hormones can accumulate. The consumption of alcohol in the U.S. has been rising steadily, and is becoming a problem for more and more women.

The importance of your liver

Your liver processes estrogen so it can be safely eliminated from the body. Estrogen is secreted by the ovaries in the form of estradiol, which the liver converts into two other types of estrogen called estrone and estriol. This ability to turn estradiol (the most carcinogenic estrogen) to estriol (the weakest active form of estrogen) is crucial.

The liver performs many other important functions that are essential for your health. It stores and filters the blood, secretes bile, and optimizes thyroid function. It has numerous metabolic functions including the conversion of sugar into glycogen (the form in which carbohydrates are stored in your body). It also plays a vital part in breaking down fat and using it to produce energy.

All these are very good reasons to drink alcohol in moderation. Do not drink every night; save it for weekends or special occasions and when you do indulge, don't have more than two glasses of wine or beer.

How to cut down

Thankfully, more and more people are becoming aware of the health problems associated with these addictive drinks and are turning to alternatives. However, as with all drugs, giving up can lead to withdrawal symptoms such as headaches, nausea, tiredness and depression, which are sometimes quite dramatic.

To minimize these effects, don't stop overnight. Cut down gradually, over a few weeks. Begin by substituting decaffeinated coffee for half of your total intake per day, then gradually change over until all the coffee you drink is decaffeinated. Don't stop at this point, though, because the problem goes beyond caffeine. As coffee is one of the most heavily sprayed plants in the world, you swallow high quantities of pesticides and other contaminants with every cup so you will eventually have to eliminate decaffeinated coffee as well. Also, although decaffeinated coffee does not contain caffeine, it does contain two other stimulants, theobromine and theophylline, which can still give you highs and lows and disturb your sleep. Slowly replace it with other drinks, such as herbal teas and grain coffees, and you should be able to give up coffee without feeling too miserable.

4 Animal products

These foods are a major source of saturated fats, which are linked to heart disease and stroke. They are high in protein too, and although you might have been brought up to believe that protein is important, it is possible to have too much. The body needs protein, which is the basic building block for all its cells and bones as well as the hair, skin and nails, but nearly everyone in the Western world eats far more than is necessary – we need much less than most people think.

Why? For a start, most of the amino acids that make up protein can be made in the body. Only eight out of a total of 25 amino acids are called "essential" because they must be obtained from food, so it easy to consume too much. A high protein diet is unhealthy because it can leach calcium from your bones, something to be avoided, especially at menopause. (For more information on high protein diets, see page 179.) Too much protein can also cause problems such as kidney stones and gout.

Meat
Beef, pork, lamb and game should, in my opinion, be omitted completely. Red meat has been linked to illnesses such as colon cancer and diverticulitis (a condition in which parts of the colon protrude and become inflamed). In 1997, the British government's Department of Health Committee on Medical Aspects of Food and Nutrition Policy (COMA) took the rare step of publishing a report entitled "Nutritional Aspects of the Development of Cancer," which suggested a possible link between the consumption of red meat and colon cancer and recommended that intake should be reduced to less than 3.2 ounces per day. When you consider that an average portion of bacon is 1.6 ounces while just two pork sausages weigh approximately 3.5 ounces, it makes you realize how easy it is eat far too much red meat.

Eggs
Choose organic free-range eggs, which have been produced without the use of antibiotics or other chemicals.

Dairy products
Milk, butter, cream and cheese should be eaten sparingly. Like meat, these are high in saturated fats and they can also trigger food intolerance in many people. Some people are lactose-intolerant, which means they react to the sugar milk contains, while others find that casein can aggravate skin conditions such as eczema and psoriasis. Dairy products can also cause a runny nose, excessive mucus and a feeling that you need to clear your throat.

These reactions are not surprising. After all, cow's milk is designed for calves, not humans. The cow has a four-stomach digestive system where the casein in dairy milk is dealt with efficiently. Because humans cannot digest it easily, it remains in the gut where it begins to putrefy and rot, producing toxins and mucus. The undigested matter also clings to the lining of the intestines and prevents the absorption of vital nutrients.

This digestive struggle takes a lot of energy to sort out. The energy that you would otherwise spend enjoying life and doing the things you want to do is instead being diverted to sort out your digestion and as a result, you feel tired. Of course it is very common to feel tired after a meal, particularly a heavy one, because your body is using much more energy than it should to digest the food. When you feel like that it may be worth looking at what you have eaten.

An added problem is the feed that the farmers give to their cows. Cattle can be fed antibiotics to speed their growth and increase milk yield. A generation ago, an individual cow would produce approximately 2 gallons of milk per day; now it can yield 12 gallons per day. So if you are buying dairy products, buy organic to reduce your intake of chemicals.

Of all the dairy foods, yogurt containing the cultures acidophilus or bifidus, which are found naturally in your digestive tract, are the most beneficial. They are a source of "healthy" bacteria, which can help to prevent an overgrowth of yeast in the body. When yogurt are heat-treated they lose this culture, so buy organic "live" natural yogurt. These can be marketed in different ways, so read the label carefully. "Bio" usually means "live" and "bio" yogurt will contain a culture such as lactobacillus, which will do the job. I mention organic because non-organic produce can contain antibiotics and chemicals from the animal's diet (cow's, sheep's or goat's; whatever type of milk product you choose). Fruit yogurt should be avoided because they have a very high sugar content, which can affect your blood sugar balance.

Margarine or butter?

If you reach for margarine because you want to avoid the saturated fat in butter, think again. Although margarine is manufactured from polyunsaturated fats, these "good" fats become "trans fats" in the process of hydrogenation, which makes a fat more solid and spreadable. Hydrogenated vegetable oil is listed in the ingredients of most margarines and many fast foods, such as potato chips, cookies and crackers, and the trans-fats, or trans-fatty acids, thus created have been linked to all sorts of problems, including an increased rate of heart attack and an inability to absorb essential fats.[7]

In addition, trans fats have a plastic-like quality that makes your body struggle to eliminate them. So why pressure your body to deal with a substance that you do not really need to eat? Surely it is better to make things easy for your body so that it functions efficiently and has the resources to heal itself? For this reason, I recommend using butter in moderation, organic if possible, or unhydrogenated margarine.

5 Salt

Sodium (salt) is a mineral that affects blood pressure and water retention. Where blood pressure is concerned, the equation is simple: the higher the level of sodium in your blood, the higher your blood pressure. Water balance is more complicated because potassium works with sodium to regulate your body's fluid levels and normalize your heart's rhythm. The more sodium you consume, the more potassium you need to counteract this effect. In order to achieve a healthy balance you should reduce substances that make you lose potassium, such as alcohol, coffee, sugar, diuretics and laxatives, keep your blood sugar stable and cut down on salt.

Table salt (sodium chloride) is a major source of sodium in the body. It is estimated that the average intake in the West is 10 to 20 times greater than necessary. Although salt is found naturally in all fruits, vegetables and grains, it is frequently added to food during cooking and at the table and is abundant in most convenience and prepared foods, including ketchup, salad dressings, burgers, french fries, cookies and pizzas. Even more sodium is put into your body through sodium nitrate, the preservative used in meat, and monosodium glutamate, a flavor enhancer used extensively in convenience and Chinese food. So if you do want to use salt, do so sparingly and choose sea salt or rock salt rather than table salt, which contains chemicals to make it flow freely.

How to cut down on salt

Eat more:
• freshly prepared foods, so you know what your meals contain
• herbs, garlic, ginger, lemon juice, tamari (wheat-free soy sauce) and miso in cooking to add flavor
Eat less:
• salt (especially table salt), added at the table or in cooking
• convenience foods or frozen dinners with a high salt content. Read labels carefully.

---

6 Additives

Manufacturers argue that additives, preservatives and flavorings are used in such small quantities that they will not have any adverse effects on your health. However, when you take into account the different products you eat and drink every day, these small amounts add up. They also create a chemical cocktail inside the body and nobody knows how the different elements will react with each other.

In my view, additives should be avoided entirely, although admittedly, this can be difficult. We all lead busy lives, so just do the best you can. Generally, the longer the ingredients list, the more suspicious you should be about the "naturalness" of a food. If you do need to buy convenience or packaged food, choose a quality brand and go for the one with the fewest chemicals in the list of ingredients.

The good food guide

Rather than buying food packed with additives and preservatives, make the best of the natural goodness in food.
• Organic carrots and potatoes don't need to be peeled. Just scrub them to remove the dirt because many of the nutrients are concentrated just under the skin.
• Cook vegetables lightly in a little water or steam.
• Avoid frying where possible. Try grilling or baking instead.

continued

• Choose cookware with care. Avoid aluminum cookware as this is a toxic heavy metal that can enter food through cooking. The same applies to aluminum foil and cases.
• Avoid any non-stick or coated cookware, which are thought to be carcinogenic. The best choices are cast iron pans, enamel, glass and stainless steel.

7 GM Foods

Genetic modification is an especially important subject for women, because soy, one of the most important sources of phytoestrogens, is also one of the most commonly genetically modified foods. If soy is genetically modified, it may contain fewer beneficial phytoestrogens than natural soy.[8] Up to two-thirds of processed foods contain soy, including bread, cookies, pizza and baby food, and it is thought that a high percentage of that soy has been genetically modified. Other genetically modified foods include corn, tomato paste, cheese containing chymosin (a genetically modified rennet that hardens cheese) and lecithin (which is used as an emulsifier in products such as mayonnaise), an ingredient found in many foods.

Genetic engineering is about manipulating the basic DNA, or genetic blueprint, of a plant or animal. It is this process that ensures the fittest of the species survive. This happens naturally in evolution, of course, but when nature is in charge the process is normally slow and gradual, taking hundreds of years. The argument for genetically modifying foods is that biological processes have been used for centuries to improve food supplies. This is true, but these processes did not involve transferring genes wholesale. For instance, plant breeding matches the desired characteristics of two parent-plants to create a plant that has the best features from both. To get that process right, matching may have to be done many times during many years of trial and error. The gene manipulation that humans are tinkering with now bypasses both evolution and breeding programs, and as yet we don't know what the price will be.

During the process of genetic modification, genes from other species are introduced into a plant to make it more resistant to pests, viruses or weed killers. This can make it almost impossible to avoid allergens. If a nut gene is inserted into a soybean, for example, people who are allergic to nuts will also be allergic to the soy milk or whatever other product is made from the genetically modified crop.

GM also produces alliances that would be impossible in nature. For instance, it is now possible to buy a tomato that contains a fish gene to boost its frost-resistance. The gene comes from flounder, which survive well in cold water. The same gene has also been introduced into salmon, which normally stops eating and growing in the cold dark days of winter. Adding a flounder gene prompts salmon to feed all year round, speeding up their growth rate by 400 percent. Many conservationists are concerned about what could happen if GM salmon being bred in pens escape into the wild, as well as about the immediate threat of effluent from the pens polluting coastal waters.

In order to smuggle these new genes across the species barrier, scientists use infectious agents (viruses and bacteria). Then antibiotic-resistant genes are added as genetic markers to allow the scientists to track the movements of the new genes. The British Medical Association (BMA) fears that this antibiotic resistance might transfer to animals and humans, leaving them vulnerable to disease. For example, genetically modified corn contains a marker gene that passes on resistance to ampicillin, an important antibiotic used to treat bronchitis, ear infections and urinary tract infections. As a result, the BMA has called for studies to see whether GM foods could damage the immune system or cause birth defects. There is also the possibility that resistance could be transferred to the natural bacteria in the intestine, creating lethal substances and a whole generation of diseases that could not be killed off by antibiotics. My advice is to avoid genetically modified foods where possible and buy organic. If we as consumers consciously do not buy these foods, eventually there may not be a market for them.

Admittedly, detecting GM foods can be difficult, which makes it impossible to make an informed choice about what you are buying. The best way is to read the label with care. If a food contains soy oil or lecithin, be suspicious because it does not have to be labeled "genetically modified." I used to buy my canned tuna in soy oil and have now switched to tuna in spring water for precisely this reason.

CHAPTER 7

New Thinking about Osteoporosis

You may have been told you need to take HRT "for your bones." Not every woman gets osteoporosis, however, so is it worth risking another problem such as invasive breast cancer to take a medication for a disease you may never get? And if you do decide to take HRT purely for your bones, when can you come off it? The answer is that you can't, because HRT only seems to protect the bones for as long as you take it, and your greatest risk of hip fractures starts at around 70 years of age. So if you start taking HRT at menopause you could end up taking it continuously for 30 to 50 years. If one were to take a cynical view, this would obviously seem to be in the pharmaceutical industry's interest.

Knowing whether you are at risk of developing osteoporosis will make it easier to decide if you should consider HRT or one of the other drugs specifically designed to treat the condition. You may be able to do without medication entirely. The first thing to do is to look at your risk factors and then devise a step-by-step plan to help you make decisions about what treatment, if any, is right for you.

Good bone structure

Bone consists of several different elements:

- the dense outer cortical bone, which is renewed completely every 10 to 12 years
- the inner, spongy trabecular layer, which has a faster turnover and is completely replaced every two to three years. The wrists and hips contain a large amount of trabecular bone and the most common fractures occur here. The spine also contains substantial amounts but the vertebrae are protected by their shape, which adds strength.
- a framework made up of collagen that gives flexibility, plus calcium and phosphorous crystals for strength

continued

Building bone

Keeping your bones strong depends on a number of different systems in the body. Bone is living tissue, that is constantly being broken down and replaced. Old bone is weak so this renewal, which is called remodeling, is vital for bone strength. It involves two different kinds of cells and several hormones. Bone remodeling is characterized by a process called "coupling" where old or damaged bone is dissolved by cells called osteoclasts and the new cavity is filled by new bone created by others called osteoblasts. The formation is said to be coupled, because when old bone is removed, new bone is formed at exactly the same location. In young people this is perfectly balanced, so no bone loss occurs.

Losing bone

Osteoclast cells dissolve old or damaged bone, a process called bone resorption.

Parathyroid hormone acts on the osteoclasts, which resorb bone. If blood levels of calcium drop, parathyroid hormone, manufactured by the parathyroid glands, takes calcium from the bones and circulates it in the blood to correct the imbalance. It also stops calcium being flushed out via the urine and activates vitamin D so that you absorb more calcium from your food. So if your body registers that you do not have enough calcium or vitamin D from what you are eating, you could be losing bone density.

Restoring bone

Osteoblast cells fill the cavities left by removal of the old bone. This is called bone formation.

Calcium is incorporated into the bones by the action of a hormone called calcitonin, produced by the thyroid gland, which acts on the osteoblasts to help build new bone. Ninety-nine percent of your body's calcium is stored in your bones and teeth and in addition to calcitonin, you need both stomach (hydrochloric) acid (see page 87) and vitamin D in order to absorb it properly.

The sex hormones also play an important part in renewing bone. Estrogen stops the production of parathyroid hormone that removes calcium from the bones and stimulates the release of bone-building calcitonin. Testosterone triggers the osteoblasts and increases levels of the enzyme that helps to form calcium crystals in the bone.

continued

Although estrogen production in the ovaries slows dramatically at menopause, sex hormones are also secreted by the adrenal glands. These produce small amounts of estrogen and testosterone plus a substance called androstenedione, which is converted to a form of estrogen by body fat.

So you can see how many of the body's processes are interrelated and that keeping your bones healthy is not just a case of taking extra calcium in your diet or swallowing calcium supplements.

The osteoporosis puzzle

Osteoporosis is often called a "silent disease" because there may not be any symptoms at all. But it can be argued that osteoporosis (which, after all, is only the label given to bone mineral density that falls below a threshold arbitrarily defined by the World Health Organization) is essentially a risk factor for fractures. Osteoporosis is a warning that your bones may be liable to break, just as high blood pressure (hypertension) is a warning that you are at higher risk of experiencing a stroke or heart attack. It is just one of a number of important factors, such as diet and exercise, that need attention.

Women reach their peak bone density around the age of 25, which is why it is important for young women to be active and build up a good bone density before that age. The higher your peak bone density, the lower your risk of osteoporosis in later life. Studies show that women who have good bone density at the age of 50 have a negligible risk of hip fracture later in life while those who already have osteoporosis by that age have a 50 percent risk of having a hip fracture as they get older.[1] Even so, it is important to remember that 50 percent of women diagnosed with osteoporosis at 50 do not get a hip fracture when they are older. It is still a 50:50 chance.

Bone density is only part of the story, however, because bone turnover – the rate at which bone is dissolved and renewed – is crucial too. The bone loss that happens around the time of menopause, when levels of protective estrogen drop, occurs because more cavities are created, making the bone more fragile. (This is important because the strength of bone lies in its structure.) This may be because the process of bone renewal changes, increasing the rate of bone turnover. One of two things can happen. Either there is more activity generally, so bone is dissolved and formed at an increased rate, resulting in a loss of bone density of up to 5 percent a year, or else more bone is removed than is laid down.

Not every woman experiences a dramatic loss of bone after menopause, however. As part of the well-known PEPI (Postmenopausal Estrogen/Progestin Interventions) Trial to investigate the impact of HRT on bone density, researchers found that 40 percent of the women who were not taking HRT during the three-month trial had stable bones. They did not experience bone loss at the spine or hip,[2] yet some women who were taking HRT still lost bone.

Everybody loses bone over time – it is part of the normal aging process. This slower, age-related bone loss is caused by reduced activity of the bone-building cells. It is experienced by both sexes, but can have a disproportionate effect on women, who live longer than men and have a longer time in which to succumb to fractures. Women also tend to have smaller bones anyway.

Osteoporosis occurs when bone loss becomes excessive and the bones become filled with tiny pores, or holes, which make them increasingly fragile. The first sign is often a fracture caused by a minor accident, such as twisting your ankle while walking or stubbing a toe. At present it is estimated that 40 in 100 women will experience one or more fractures after the age of 50, usually of the hip, spine or forearm.[3] Men suffer from osteoporosis too, although their lifetime risk is only 6 percent for a hip fracture compared to 17.5 percent for women.[4]

There is still much to find out about osteoporosis and the current rise in the number of cases may be due to causes other than the drop in hormones at menopause and the effect of a lengthening lifespan on our bones. There is some evidence that it could be a modern phenomenon, triggered by diet and lifestyle. In 1993, *The Lancet* published the results of the examination of some 18th-century remains of a number of women, which were discovered beneath a church. The bones were from Caucasian women (who are now thought to be more at risk of osteoporosis) aged between 15 and 89, but studies showed that they were stronger and denser than the bones of any modern women, either pre-menopausal or post-menopausal.[5] Something in our modern lifestyle is clearly affecting the density and strength of our bones, and only now are we beginning to understand what that might be.

Measuring osteoporosis

The World Health Organization defines osteoporosis as a "progressive systemic skeletal disease characterized by low bone mass and microarchitectural deterioration of bone tissue, with a consequent increase in bone fragility and susceptibility to fracture."[6] It also divides

continued

bone into three categories marked by "standard deviations" – units of variation used in statistics – from the average peak bone density found in healthy young women. These are:
- Normal – less than one standard deviation below the average for young women.
- Osteopenia – when bone density is low but is not severe enough to be classed as osteoporosis – between one and 2.5 standard deviations below.
- Osteoporosis – lower than 2.5 standard deviations below.

Are you at risk?

You can assess your chances of having osteoporosis by checking out the factors that increase your risk. It's important to remember that these don't mean that you are destined to have osteoporosis. Although you cannot alter your history or your genetic make-up, there is a lot you can do to change your diet and lifestyle that can help to strengthen your bones.

1. Your mother had osteoporosis
You probably know that if your mother (or even your father) had osteoporosis, you are at higher risk. The condition may not have been diagnosed, so consider whether anyone in the family had any obvious signs, such as a dowager's hump (an outward curving of the spine known medically as kyphosis) or lost height as they aged, because the bones in the spine were being compressed or crushed. Keep an eye on your own height too. Do you now have to stand on tiptoe to reach a cupboard which you could reach easily before?

It's worth investigating your family history because new research emphasizes the link between heredity and osteoporosis. Recent studies of identical twins suggest that as much as 75 to 80 percent of bone development may be genetically determined. Identical twins have exactly the same genes, so it is possible to isolate the impact of heredity from the effects of lifestyle and the environment. Unlike fraternal, or non-identical twins, whose genes (and bones) show no more similarities than you would expect between ordinary brothers and sisters, identical twins of both sexes and all ages have almost the same bone mineral density.

The studies suggest that the genes regulating bone density influence both peak bone mass (when bones are at their strongest) and the rate at which bone is lost. It is probable that more than one gene may be involved. Different "candidate genes" as they are called are being investigated to pinpoint those that control how the body uses vitamin D, and to find out if others can prevent the absorption of estrogen or are involved in collagen metabolism, a major bone protein. Scientists are now working on a blood test to identify people who carry a mutation of the COLIA1 gene, which regulates collagen metabolism. A four-year pilot study has shown that picking up this genetic marker in the blood can predict fractures as effectively as bone scanning.

2. You are of European or Asian descent

Your ethnic origin also makes a difference to your risk of developing osteoporosis. Although osteoporosis is common among Asian and Caucasian women, African women seem to be relatively immune. There are variations within racial groups too, because women from Northern Europe are more at risk than those from Mediterranean countries. So why the difference? It is probably caused by differences in peak bone mass or maximum bone density, which is acquired in early life. The greater this is, the more protection women have against bone loss at menopause. A number of factors can affect it. On the downside, an inactive lifestyle, combined with a lack of sunlight, which depresses the production of vitamin D, could explain the higher incidence of osteoporosis in women from Northern Europe. Afro-Caribbean women, on the other hand, may have natural protection. It is known that they are more susceptible to fibroids, benign growths in the uterus that are known to be sensitive to estrogen. If Afro-Caribbean women are producing higher levels of estrogen than Asian or Caucasian women, they may have an inbuilt resistance to osteoporosis.

3. You have had an eating disorder

Women who have suffered or are suffering from anorexia or bulimia should be aware that they are at increased risk of osteoporosis. The reduction in body fat that follows a restricted diet can put a stop to periods and also affects the bones. It used to be thought that the bone loss experienced by women who suffered from anorexia was a direct result of reduced estrogen production, which depends on a certain percentage of body fat, but it now seems that estrogen deficiency may not be the cause. Research into bone loss in young women with anorexia nervosa and athletic women whose periods have stopped seems to show that rather than breaking down bone faster than they are building it, as is often the case around menopause, these women are simply not building up enough bone in the first place.[7] It seems that the "energy deficit" caused by their restricted food intake affects bone formation and causes metabolic changes, including problems with thyroid hormones and insulin, which interfere with bone formation. Interestingly, these women do not seem to have any problems with calcium-regulating hormones, so that cannot be responsible for the bone loss.[8] However, any woman who has been restricting food intake for some time is likely to be deficient in nutrients such as calcium, magnesium and zinc, which are essential for bone health. My recommendation is that if you suffer from an eating disorder you should ask for a bone density scan (see page 89) and do a bone turnover test (see page 90). You should also have a bone scan and a bone turnover test if you had an eating disorder when you were younger but have been healthy for a number of years because your past medical history may put you more at risk of developing osteoporosis later on in life.

4. Your periods have been irregular
If you have experienced irregular cycles or missed periods for several months before you reached menopause, you will have lost the protective effect of those circulating female hormones for some time. Women with a history of irregular periods before the age of 40 have an average loss in bone density of more than 8 percent compared to women with regular periods.[9]

5. You are (or were) a smoker
Smoking can reduce bone density by up to 25 percent. Not only does it reduce bone density, it also increases the risk of hip fractures.[10] In addition, smoking alters the profile of female hormones, which can trigger an earlier menopause, reducing levels of the estrogen that helps to protect your bones.[11]

6. You have taken medication that affects your bones
Because some drugs accelerate bone loss, it is important to check the effect of any medication you are taking (or have taken) long term. The drugs that can increase your risk of osteoporosis include:

• Steroid medication (oral corticosteroids such as prednisolone) prescribed for chronic inflammatory disorders such as rheumatoid arthritis or ulcerative colitis. Corticosteroids cause a reduction in bone formation that can result in a 10 to 15 percent overall bone loss and make fractures more likely.[12] Although it is often said that inhaled steroids, taken by people with asthma, have no impact on the bones, new research shows that the more puffs per day a woman takes, the greater her bone loss.[13] So it is important that if you use or have used inhaled steroids, you should have your bone density checked (see page 89). Make sure that you follow a bone-friendly diet (see page 98), exercise well (see page 106) and take extra nutrients in the form of food supplements as recommended on page 99.

• Laxatives and diuretics. Regular use can put you at increased risk of osteoporosis because calcium and other essential nutrients may be excreted from the body.

• Drugs for thyroid problems. It has been known for many years that there is a link between overactive thyroid (hyperthyroidism or thyrotoxicosis) and osteoporosis.[14] This condition is characterized by high levels of thyroid hormones, which cause low absorption of calcium, low levels of parathyroid hormone that play an essential role in bone formation (see page 184) and a subsequent increase in bone turnover. You could also be at increased risk of osteoporosis if you have been taking thyroid hormone for an underactive thyroid (hypothyroidism) at too high a dose for many years. That is why it is important to have your levels monitored to make sure that you are taking the appropriate amount.

• The blood-thinning drug, heparin, which is increasingly used to prevent miscarriage.

If you are unlucky enough to suffer from osteoporosis as a result of taking prescription medicine, it is worth knowing that treatment is available with bisphosphonates (antiresorptive drugs – see page 91).

7. *You don't get much exercise*

Bone gains strength from the demands made on it: you use it or you lose it as far as protection against osteoporosis is concerned. These demands come from the force gravity exerts on your bones and the way your muscles contract, which also helps to maintain bone density. The absence of gravity is the reason why astronauts lose some of their bone density while up in space. Nature is very logical. Why maintain bone density when a gravity-free environment means that the body does not have to support itself?

The exercise needed to keep your bones strong should be the load-bearing kind that exerts pressure on the bones, and the best forms are described in Chapter 12. The good news is that it needn't be excessive. Even moderate exercise can help to increase bone density in women after menopause. By keeping yourself fit you also improve your coordination and flexibility, which makes you less likely to fall, and that, in turn, reduces the risk of fractures.

8. *You exercise too much*

Exercising to extremes can be as much of a problem as not exercising enough. Nature always favors a balance and just as it is not healthy to be under- or overweight, so it can be damaging to exercise too much or too little.

Women who are involved in intense physical training, such as athletics or ballet dancing, often find that their periods stop because they have lost too much body fat. This puts them at risk of osteoporosis, so while it is essential to exercise, it is important not to overdo it.

9. You are underweight

Women are under a lot of pressure from the media to be ultra-slim, but conforming to this ideal can put your bones at risk, especially at menopause. Although your ovaries reduce the production of estrogen at this time, your fat cells continue to produce a weak form of estrogen called estrone. A certain amount of body fat is necessary for the adequate production of estrone, which can help to protect against osteoporosis.

Of course, health risks come with being overweight, but it is also important to avoid being underweight. We know that African women have a very small risk of developing osteoporosis and maybe this is because a super-slim body shape is not desirable in their culture, so dieting is a rarity.

10. You had an early menopause

Some women experience menopause before the age of 40 for no known reason, but premature menopause (usually considered to be before the age of 40) can also be caused by radiotherapy given to treat cancer or by surgical removal of the ovaries. If menopause is brought on by radiotherapy or surgery, estrogen levels drop quickly instead of declining gradually, as is normal during menopause. This sudden drop can cause a very rapid rate of bone loss for about five years after the treatment.

11. You have problems with your digestion

For your body to absorb the nutrients essential to keep your bones strong, your digestive system needs to work efficiently. Among the problems that may arise are:

• Insufficient stomach (hydrochloric) acid. As you get older you produce less stomach acid and this can interfere with the proper absorption of calcium and other nutrients. It is estimated that about 40 percent of post-menopausal women are severely deficient in stomach acid so even if you are eating well and taking supplements, you could be fighting a losing battle if you can't digest or absorb them. Frequent use of antacids for digestive problems is not good for your bones because they contain aluminum, which accelerates the excretion of calcium. It is important to sort out the reason why you are getting digestive problems rather than just take indigestion tablets when you get symptoms. Laboratory tests are available to assess how well your digestive system is working.

• Celiac disease. This digestive disorder is characterized by an intolerance to gluten found in grains such as wheat, rye, barley and oats. People who have coeliac disease have white blood cells in their gut lining that are programmed to "see" gluten as a foreign substance and so reject it. This causes malabsorption of a number of essential nutrients and is therefore a risk factor for osteoporosis. Many deficiencies have been noted in sufferers of coeliac disease, including insufficient levels of vitamins A, D, E, K, folic acid and other B vitamins, zinc and selenium. The disease also makes the absorption of calcium difficult, especially where there is a deficiency of vitamin D.

WHAT SCREENING CAN (AND CAN'T) DO

It is important to take steps to assess the strength of your bones if you have any of the risk factors listed above. A bone density scan and a bone turnover test, for example, will give you the information you need and allow you to make choices according to what is most appropriate for you. If you discover that your bones are more fragile than they should be, you can do something about it before it becomes a major problem.

If all is well, the bone density scan will show that your bones are strong. In this case, especially if you find that you can control the symptoms of menopause naturally, why take HRT? I believe that healthy women with healthy bones simply don't need unnecessary intervention, and that any benefits of HRT are simply not worth the risk.

If you find out that your bone density is less than it should be (osteopenia) then you can work on making the changes needed to prevent the development of full-blown osteoporosis. Because bone density can be measured and monitored, you can continue to assess your bone strength, and if the situation changes and your bone density becomes a matter for concern, you can always change your mind about treatment. However, if the diagnosis is osteoporosis rather than osteopenia, you should take action straight away, and consider a more conventional form of treatment.

It is important to remember that there are limitations to bone density scans. I have seen 50-year-old women who have returned from their doctors with a "diagnosis" of osteoporosis made from a bone density scan, terrified because they have been told they have the bones of an 80-year-old and should not even lift a suitcase. But it could be that some women have constitutionally low bone density, and not a condition that has been caused by menopause. Nobody knows what a scan taken at the age of 25 (when peak bone mass is reached) would have shown. If bone density was very low then, there might have been little change over the past 15 years. Post-menopausal Chinese women, for example, have significantly lower hip bone mineral density than Caucasian women and are in theory at higher risk of osteoporosis.[15] Yet they have fewer fractures, probably because they have a lower rate of bone loss, which suggests that their rate of turnover is lower.

Another problem is that although scans can assess bone density they cannot predict who will have a fracture. An article in the *British Medical Journal* published in 1999 asked why doctors continued to measure bone density when analysis of 11 separate studies and over 2000 fractures concluded that the scans "cannot identify individuals who will have a fracture."[16] The author argued that it may be more appropriate to measure bone turnover – the rate at which bone is lost – rather than bone density, because bone is a living dynamic tissue. "Bone depends for strength more on its architecture than on its mass," the article went on. "If a bolt or two at a time were removed from a cantilever bridge for replacement, architectural strength might not be affected – but if a thousand were removed at one time (a high turnover state) architectural strength could be compromised critically, with little loss of mass."

So the best way to measure bone health is a combination of a bone density scan and bone turnover analysis. They measure your bones in two different ways, and together provide valuable information. A qualified practitioner can then help you to plan your best course of action depending on the results of both of these.

TESTING FOR OSTEOPOROSIS
These are the tests most commonly used to assess your bone status.

1. The DEXA Scan (Dual Energy X-ray Absorptiometry)
This test is the gold standard for measuring bone density. It is administered by a scanner that uses two simultaneous X-ray energy beams – one high-energy and the other low-energy. The low-energy beam can pass through soft tissue but not bone so your bone density can be calculated by working out the difference between the two readings. The scanner can measure bone mineral density at many different points on the body. This is important because density at one part of the body does not necessarily reflect the situation at other points. With osteoporosis, bone loss typically starts in the trabecular bones (such as the spine and hip), so these are important sites to test.

A DEXA scan does have some drawbacks. One is that you are exposing yourself to X-rays. However, only a low dose of radiation is involved and as the scan is usually repeated no sooner than every two years (rarely after one) the risks are negligible when set against the benefits of obtaining an accurate snapshot of your bones.

Another disadvantage is that although both hip and spine are measured during a DEXA scan, there can be difficulties estimating the strength of your spine. This is because conditions such as osteoarthritis and scoliosis, which is curvature of the spine, can give falsely high readings of bone mineral density.[17]

2. Bone Turnover Analysis
It is possible to measure bone turnover by measuring the biochemical markers present in blood or urine. Some of these assess the rate at which bone is dissolved and others gauge the speed at which it is replaced. Two of the markers that monitor the rate at which bone is broken down, N-telopeptide (NTx) and deoxypyridinoline, can be measured in urine. At the moment NTx seems to be the more sensitive and specific, especially in women.[18] It is sufficiently accurate to predict the risk of osteoporotic fracture independently, without needing the back-up of a bone mineral density scan.[19]

Because bone turnover analysis can be repeated regularly (six-monthly is the norm) it can be helpful in monitoring treatment. If you decide to take HRT and/or start exercising and/or take supplements, this test can tell you whether your treatment is working. There are some women who do not respond to HRT or drugs for osteoporosis, and if this is picked up by a simple urine test, then another course of treatment can be suggested and time is not wasted taking something that isn't effective. Also, if you have been making changes in your diet and lifestyle, it is helpful to see that what you are doing is working since this can give you the motivation to keep going.

3. Quantitative Ultrasound
In this procedure, sound waves are passed through the heel bone (calcaneus) which, like the hip and spine, is rich in trabecular bone, to provide information about bone density. It is not as precise as the DEXA scan and it cannot measure the usual site of osteoporotic fracture, the hip. Additionally, there is no single standard for ultrasound machines, so different makes can give different results. In some studies, however, ultrasound of the heel has been shown to predict future hip fractures in older women (75 years and over),[20] so it may have more value for a certain section of the population.

The other criticism is that ultrasound devices do not actually measure bone mineral density (on which the WHO definition of osteoporosis is based) but derive information from other factors related to bone strength such as stiffness and elasticity. The British National Osteoporosis Society's (NOS) official position on the use of ultrasound is that because it "does not measure bone mineral content or density directly, it cannot be used to diagnose osteoporosis as currently defined."[21] But because ultrasound is portable and relatively inexpensive, the NOS suggests it could be used to decide which women should go for a DEXA scan.

Drug treatment for osteoporosis

HORMONE REPLACEMENT THERAPY

HRT is often prescribed on the grounds that by raising estrogen levels, it will protect your bones. Whether HRT can actually prevent fractures (and contrary to popular opinion, it does not always do this) is discussed on page 36. I'd simply like to reiterate that because the greatest risk of hip and wrist fractures in women is around the age of 75, HRT may not be required until that time. In fact, you may not need it at all. It is important to remember that pharmaceutical companies have a stake in the early use of HRT. If you begin this form of treatment in your mid-40s, you will have many years of "paying out." Don't fall into that trap. If you choose HRT, consider the reasons carefully, and remember that unless your tests show otherwise, bone loss will not be an issue until much later in your life.

The enormous revolution in testing procedures means that your bone density and bone turnover can be assessed regularly. Because it is now much easier to assess whether or not you are at risk of osteoporosis, you have every reason to postpone your decision about HRT until much later. Why wait? Because HRT is associated with a host of health problems, such as an increased risk of breast cancer, heart disease and stroke, and there is no need to risk these if you don't need to do so. Is it logical to take HRT to prevent osteoporosis, which may not happen until you are 70 or 80, but which could cause breast cancer or thrombosis in your 50s or 60s?

BISPHOSPHONATES

Bisphosphonates were originally used in industry as water softeners and antiscaling agents, since they prevented the formation of calcium carbonate crystals. Now they are the non-hormonal "anti-resorptive" drugs, specifically used to treat osteoporosis. The drugs most commonly used are Etridonate (Didronel) and alendronate (Fosamax) and risedronate (Actonel). They work by inhibiting osteoclast activity, which means they reduce the rate at which bone is broken down. These drugs will maintain bone density for as long as they are continued and are effective at reducing the risk of fracture however old you are when you start to take them. Although they do not restore lost bone, they can prevent further loss and can halve the risk of fracture in osteoporotic bones, although unfortunately that protection is rapidly lost when they are stopped.[22]

Etridonate (Didronel) has been available for more than 30 years. Taking it involves a complicated regime because you cannot eat for two hours before and two hours after swallowing the tablets. This is because the drug is poorly absorbed and any food or other vitamins and minerals taken at the same time could prevent it from working. An additional problem is that etridronate has to be taken in cycles of 14 days followed by 76 days on a calcium formulation. This on-off procedure has to be followed because etridronate binds to bone and can affect bone mineralization. Taking it continuously and in high doses as it was 20 years ago can result in soft bones (osteomalacia).

Luckily the newer bisphosphonates, alendronate and risedronate, do not seem to cause this problem when taken continuously alendronate (Fosamax) is 700 times more potent than etidronate[23] but can reduce the likelihood of fractures by 40–50 percent.[24] Risedronate (Actonel), the latest bisphosphonate, is licensed to prevent osteoporosis in women at high risk of the disease and to reduce the likelihood of spinal damage in postmenopausal women who have already had a fracture. It is 1,000 times more potent than etidronate and has been shown to increase bone mineral density and to reduce most fractures by 39 percent over three years.[25]

Unfortunately, all bisphosphonates have side-effects, including digestive disturbances. Alendronate seems to be the worst offender, so you are told to take it on an empty stomach and then remain upright for at least 30 minutes because it irritates the esophagus (the tube leading to the stomach). To minimize the problem, it is now possible to take alendronate as a once-weekly treatment, although all the previous precautions still have to be followed.

SODIUM FLUORIDE

This is a real hot potato. Fluoride is an approved osteoporosis treatment in several countries, including France and Germany (although not the U.S. or the U.K.), because it is said to be the only agent that can directly stimulate bone formation. All other treatments for osteoporosis are antiresorptive – in other words, they just stop bone being lost. But although studies suggest that fluoride triggers large increases in bone density, nobody knows whether this new bone is strong enough and current evidence suggests that there is not a subsequent reduction in fractures. As the British Department of Health's Committee on the Medical Aspects of Food (COMA) has pointed out, the incorporation of fluoride into bone disturbs the alignment of the crystals, making the bone structurally weak and even more fragile than the existing bones. Side-effects from the treatment include gastric irritation, vomiting and pain in the legs.

What about fluoride in the water? In the U.S., most of the water supply is artificially fluoridated to 2 parts per million. When it occurs naturally, fluoride is derived from the minerals the water passes through and occurs at levels of around 0.1 to 2 parts per million. High levels can increase the risk of hip fractures.[26]

The highest dose of fluoride you are likely to get comes from toothpaste, where it can reach extremely high levels of 1,000 ppm. Excess fluoride cannot cause tooth loss because unlike bone, enamel and dentine are not constantly being broken down and built up again, but it can lead to dental fluorosis, where the teeth are visibly pitted and stained. (Of course, there could be problems if swallowed in excess amounts.)

CALCITONIN

Calcitonin is a hormone produced by cells in the thyroid gland that prevents the breakdown of bone. It is available as a nasal spray. It used to be available only in the form of a daily injection, to be used on a short-term basis. The nasal spray is licensed for the treatment of established osteoporosis in post-menopausal women and is known to reduce the risk of fractures. The most common side effect of using the nasal spray is rhinitis (runny nose).

The nutritional approach to healthy bones

Everyone can benefit from an eating plan that concentrates on foods and supplements to boost bone health, but it is just as important to avoid the substances that can weaken your bones. The aim is to look at your diet and to eliminate any foods or drink that will have a negative effect.

If you have any risk factors for osteoporosis or have been told that your bone density is low, then the foods and drinks listed here should be eliminated or kept to a minimum. Even if you do not have osteoporosis and your bones are normal, or a little below, it is worth following the recommendations set out here, so that you can maintain that good bone density or prevent a minor problem from becoming a major one. The same applies if you already have osteoporosis. Of course you will need some medical treatment, but don't write off the natural approach. Follow the advice given here alongside your treatment, so that you give your body the best chance of strengthening of your bones.

What not to eat or drink

Foods and drinks to avoid or reduce to prevent osteoporosis

- Soft, fizzy drinks
- High intake of animal protein
- Caffeine
- Sugar
- Alcohol
- Salt
- Bran
- Spinach and rhubarb

1. Soft, fizzy drinks

Fizzy drinks contain high levels of phosphorus, a mineral women should treat with caution. Why? Because when phosphorous levels in your blood rise, a message is sent to your brain telling it that there is not enough calcium. The result is that your body draws calcium from your bones and teeth to balance the high levels of phosphorus, and if this happens regularly, your bones will begin to weaken.

One major concern is that women reach their peak bone mass by the age of 25 and bone density starts to decline after that. So if young women and teenagers over-indulge in fizzy soft drinks, there is a real possibility of an osteoporosis epidemic in years to come. Colas, often a favorite with teenagers, are particularly high in phosphorous. Fizzy water, without any flavoring, is fine but fruit juices should be substituted for soft drinks, which will contain sugar (or glucose), artificial sweeteners and/or colorings.

Women of menopausal age and older should avoid soft, fizzy drinks entirely. In one study, postmenopausal women with osteoporosis were given phosphorus at each meal for 12 months.[27] The subsequent bone biopsies revealed that while bone-forming surfaces had decreased, bone-dissolving surfaces increased. This means that the phosphorus was increasing bone turnover, causing more bone to be broken down than was being restored.

2. Protein

Protein is a vital part of the diet because it is the basic building block for all the cells and bones as well as the hair, skin and nails. It is made from 25 amino acids, eight of which are called "essential" because they must be obtained from food, unlike the other 17 that can be made in the body. But too much protein can be harmful because it causes an acidic reaction that needs calcium to neutralize it. When you eat too much protein, your reserves of calcium, contained in your bones and teeth, are summoned to correct the imbalance. The calcium is then eliminated from the body through your urine, and this can eventually damage your bones.[28]

So how much protein is too much? Scientists at the Harvard School of Public Health have investigated the ideal quantities of protein in the diet. They found that women who ate more than 3.35 ounces of animal protein a day had an increased risk of forearm fractures compared with women who ate less than 2.75 ounces per day. It's interesting that women who ate vegetable rather than animal protein had no increased risk of fractures, no matter how much protein they ate.[29] In fact, studies have shown that vegetarians have greater bone density in later life. Although that may not be the case under the age of about 40, it seems that vegetarians lose bone much more slowly than meat-eaters as they age,[30] and have a lower risk of osteoporosis.[31]

Unfortunately for the state of women's bones, one of the most popular weight-loss diets is currently the high protein diet. This craze has swept the U.S., publicized by celebrities who swear by its ability to promote quick weight loss. Yet in the long term, this type of diet is not only unhealthy, but can also be dangerous.

The regime encourages you to eat lots of protein, such as meat and eggs, but few carbohydrates. Even fruit intake is strictly limited because of its carbohydrate status. The theory is that sweet and starchy foods make blood sugar levels rise sharply, prompting a surge of insulin to compensate. As mentioned on page 65, when insulin is raised, more of your food is converted into fat, and you begin to put on weight. So it is believed that by cutting out anything that prevents a surge of insulin, you will lose weight.

It sounds logical, and it can cause dramatic weight loss. When the body is starved of carbohydrates, it looks for energy in its glycogen stores. Because 4 grams (0.14 ounce) of water clings to every gram of glycogen, it is possible to lose a lot of weight very quickly – but initially this is water, not fat. Only when the glycogen stores are depleted does the body start to dissolve fat.

A high-protein diet has two potentially harmful effects quite apart from the damage it can do to your bones. The first is that it can cause an abnormal metabolic state called ketosis, because there is not enough carbohydrate stored in the liver for the body to use. Ketones accumulate in the blood, causing side-effects such as bad breath (there is a fruity odor of acetone on the breath), poorer concentration, mood swings and bad memory. These symptoms are also experienced in cases of starvation and diabetes, and they are not something you would want to experience.

Secondly, this diet also causes a buildup of nitrogen in the body. Nitrogen is a byproduct of protein and is normally efficiently dealt with by the liver and kidneys, after which it is excreted through the urine. When the protein content of the diet is very high, excess nitrogen accumulates and can damage the liver and kidneys. There are healthy ways to find your natural weight, and these are explained in chapter 11 and in my book *Natural Alternatives to Dieting*.

3. *Caffeine, sugar and alcohol*

I have put these together because they have a similar effect on your bones. They all cause extreme changes in blood sugar levels which in turn stimulate the release of adrenaline. This is important because it is vital not to make demands on your adrenal glands around the time of menopause. Eventually they will be called upon to produce a form of estrogen, which can help to protect your bones once your ovaries begin to produce less.

In addition, coffee and sugar cause an acidic reaction similar to that triggered by protein and have the same effect of leaching calcium from your bones. It is possible to induce osteoporosis in hamsters if they are fed on a sugar-laden diet,[32] and we now know that drinking more than two cups of coffee a day can significantly increase the risk of hip fractures.[33]

Tea also contains caffeine, although not as much as coffee, so the acidic effect is reduced. Take care not to drink it at mealtimes because the tannin in tea binds to important minerals such as calcium and zinc and prevents their absorption in the digestive tract. Leave a gap of at least one hour before or after eating if you are going to have a cup of regular tea.

Some research, however, has shown that women who drink tea can have a higher bone density than those who do not.[34] This could be due to the flavonoid content of the tea, which has an antioxidant effect. We have seen that antioxidants can protect the body's cells from harmful free radicals (see page 56), which are linked to age-related diseases like cancer and heart disease. Less well known is the theory that antioxidants also decrease bone density.[35] However, black tea can cause fluctuations in blood sugar (see page 65) which can affect your mood, so it is better to get the antioxidants from fruits and vegetables. Green tea may be drunk in moderation, as it has stronger antioxidant effects than black, but it still contains some caffeine. Therefore, it's best to keep it to a minimum and to drink herbal teas, such as peppermint, instead.

Alcohol also contributes to osteoporosis because it acts as a diuretic, leaching out valuable minerals such as calcium and magnesium. This increases bone loss and the incidence of fractures.[36]

4. Salt
A diet high in salt (sodium) will increase calcium loss through the urine.[37] Salt is sodium chloride, which is often found in high amounts in processed and convenience foods, especially no-fat and low-fat foods. These tend to be high in both salt and sugar, which are needed to make them palatable.

5. Dairy foods
Many women increase their intake of dairy foods to fend off osteoporosis, but this can be counterproductive. Remember that milk is an animal protein, so you may be excreting more calcium than you are taking in if you eat too many dairy products. Ironically, although skimmed and two-percent milk have a lower fat content than full-fat milk, their protein levels are proportionately higher. As it is the protein that causes calcium loss via the urine, you could end up losing more calcium than you take in.

You might be interested to learn that breast-fed babies absorb more calcium from their mothers' milk than from cows' milk, despite the fact that cows' milk contains four times the amount of calcium. What is crucial is how your body uses the calcium, and many people believe that our systems were not really designed to cope with cow's milk. That is why it's important to look at all the factors that affect bones and not just fill up with dairy foods. Dairy foods are not the only source of calcium.

6. Bran
Bran is a refined food that contains substances called phytates. These act like a magnet, attracting valuable minerals such as calcium, zinc and magnesium, which are essential for your bones and your health in general. These minerals bind to the phytates and are then excreted, along with the bran, from the digestive tract. So don't add bran to cereals. It is better to eat bran in the form that nature intended – as part of the whole grain (such as wheat or oats).

7. Spinach and rhubarb
Both spinach and rhubarb contain oxalic acid, which reacts with calcium in the digestive system and stops it from being absorbed.

Foods to boost your bones

1. Fruit and vegetables
Fruit and vegetables are packed with antioxidants that not only give protection against cancer and heart disease but can also have a beneficial effect on your bones. People who eat a high intake of fruit and vegetables have been shown to maintain a good bone mineral density.[38] It is thought that this is caused by the alkaline effect produced by eating these foods, unlike the acidic reaction created by animal protein.

2. Cider vinegar
There is some interesting research into the effect of adding cider vinegar to foods. It seems that vinegar can increase calcium absorption. My recommendation would be to use cider vinegar, either in salad dressings and so on, or as a drink – just sip 1 tablespoon of cider vinegar and honey in a cupful of warm water up to three times a day.

3. Phytoestrogens
We know that the incidence of osteoporosis and hip fracture after menopause is significantly lower in Japanese women than women from Western countries,[39] and that women taking isoflavone-rich soy protein have experienced a significant improvement in bone density.[40] So include plenty of phytoestrogens such as chickpeas, lentils and soy in your diet (see page 48).

4. Herbs
Herbs rich in calcium and other minerals are often used alongside other methods in the long-term treatment of osteoporosis. A combination of dried herbs can be made into a herbal tea and drunk on a regular basis. If you have any of the risk factors for osteoporosis or have been told you have low bone density, take a cupful each day.

The best herbs to choose (and you can blend these together) are alfalfa herb (*Medicago sativa*), nettles (*Urtica spp.*) and horsetail (*Equisetum arvense*), a natural source of silica. In animal studies, silicon prevented the loss of bone in rats whose ovaries had been removed, and it has been suggested that silicon may reduce the rate at which bone is broken down while increasing the rate at which it is formed.[41]

Supplements for bone health

The first supplement that comes to mind to combat osteoporosis is calcium. There's no doubt that calcium is important to build up and maintain the strength of the bones, but high levels in your diet or in supplements are no guarantee that the calcium is actually being absorbed. Calcium needs both stomach acid and vitamin D in order to be effective. Many other nutrients are equally crucial for healthy bones, and these include magnesium, vitamin C vitamin D, zinc and the mineral boron. This is why it is important not to focus exclusively on calcium as a supplement for bone health, but to take a range of nutrients that are important for the bones.

VITAMIN D

Without good levels of vitamin D, you cannot absorb calcium from your food or from health supplements. You may be getting plenty of calcium in your diet, but if your body thinks there is not enough in your blood, it will begin to take it from your bones. Over time this will cause bone loss.

Vitamin D helps to regulate blood levels of both calcium and phosphorus. In the digestive system, adequate levels of vitamin D are needed to transport calcium across the wall of the intestines and to move both calcium and phosphorus into your bones.

Exposing the skin to sunlight stimulates the formation of vitamin D, which is actually a hormone. The ultraviolet rays convert a substance in the skin to a pre-vitamin D which is changed in the liver and kidneys into the active form, called calcitriol. Calcitriol maintains constant calcium levels in the blood. Unfortunately sunscreen interferes with the production of this vitamin. I think the current recommendations that everyone should stay out of the sun or use a very strong sunscreen are too extreme. For example, the Environmental Protection Agency now advises that sunlight could be so dangerous that we should "protect ourselves against ultraviolet light whenever we can see our shadow."[42] Sunlight in moderation is fine, as long as you are sensible and avoid the hottest part of the day. You need some exposure to the sun in order to produce vitamin D through the skin to protect your bones. And the Australians are now finding that the effects of the anti-sun campaign are causing a deficiency in 1 in 4 people.

The major sources of vitamin D in the diet are from eggs and oily fish. And in the West other sources include fortified foods such as margarine and breakfast cereals. Calcium and vitamin D taken together as a supplement have been found to benefit the bones. In one study, elderly men and women who took a combination of vitamin D and calcium for three years showed increases in bone density. But when they stopped taking the supplements the effect was reversed, and within two years their bone turnover rates had returned to the level they were before taking the extra nutrients.[43]

VITAMIN C

Vitamin C manufactures collagen, a sort of "cement" that holds the bone matrix – the structure of the bone – together. As collagen makes up as much as 90 percent of the bone matrix, vitamin C has an important role in preventing osteoporosis. Collagen is important for the growth and repair of cells, gums, blood vessels and teeth as well as bones, and prevents problems such as easy bruising because it helps to strengthen blood vessels. In fact scurvy, a disease caused by vitamin C deficiency and characterized by swollen, bleeding gums followed by the opening of previously healed wounds, is actually a collagen disorder.

Your body cannot make or store vitamin C, so you have to get it from your diet. It is important that you are getting enough, and if osteoporosis is a risk factor for you, then I would suggest you also take it in supplement form.

FOLIC ACID

This B vitamin can help to protect your bones by reducing levels of homocysteine in the blood. Homocysteine comes from the breakdown of methionine, one of the essential amino acids, which should, in normal circumstances, be detoxified by the body. High homocysteine levels in menopausal women have been associated with an increase in bone loss, but giving women folic acid has helped to control them.[44]

Folic acid is present in the majority of unprocessed foods and green leafy vegetables, peas and green beans are especially rich sources. However, supplements may be needed to boost your intake. A B-complex tablet containing folic acid should be sufficient, and this will also contain vitamin B6, which is equally important for the bones. Vitamin B6 has been found to be deficient in people with hip fractures, and in animal studies, rats fed a diet low in B6 developed osteoporosis.[45]

VITAMIN K

Vitamin K is a fat-soluble vitamin made in the large intestine. It is primarily known for its role in blood-clotting, but it is also needed to make osteocalcin, a unique protein found in large amounts in bone. As osteocalcin helps to harden calcium, vitamin K is vital for healthy bones. Green vegetables (broccoli, cabbage and lettuce), whole grains and soy are important for the formation of vitamin K, and so are the beneficial bacteria in the intestine.

Frequent use of antibiotics, which can destroy these bacteria, can lead to a vitamin K deficiency, which is bad news for your bones because low levels of vitamin K have been linked both to fractures resulting from osteoporosis and low bone density.[46] Women who suffer from bowel disorders that affect absorption, such as coeliac disease, Crohn's disease, or ulcerative colitis, are especially at risk because they may not be able to maintain adequate levels of vitamin K.

MAGNESIUM

Sixty percent of your body's magnesium is contained in your bones, so magnesium is just as important as calcium in keeping osteoporosis at bay. Magnesium helps to process calcium and vitamin C and also plays a part in converting vitamin D to the active form that ensures calcium is efficiently absorbed by your body.

Magnesium is also essential for the normal function of the parathyroid gland, which releases parathyroid hormone, one of the "bone hormones." One study, which compared groups of women with and without osteoporosis, found that although none of them had low levels of calcium, the women with osteoporosis had low levels of other bone nutrients, including magnesium and zinc.[47] They also had low levels of a magnesium-dependent enzyme called alkaline phosphatase, which is an indication that the bone is not renewing itself adequately.

A good supply of magnesium is important because lack of magnesium can slow bone growth, decrease bone renewal and contribute to fragile bones.[48] If rats are given a diet where magnesium is restricted, they start to show abnormal bone turnover.[49]

Although magnesium can be obtained from dark green vegetables, apples, seeds, nuts, figs and lemons, supplements have an impressive record. The long-term use (over two years) of magnesium supplements after menopause has been shown to prevent fractures. In one trial, 71 percent of women experienced a significant increase in bone density and bone loss was halted in 16 percent.[50]

CALCIUM

Ninety-nine percent of your body's calcium is stored in your bones and teeth. So obviously you need calcium for your bones – but you also need to be able to absorb the calcium you take and that depends to a great extent on the supplement you choose. Not all forms of calcium are the same and it is much better to take a supplement containing calcium citrate than one made from calcium carbonate.

Calcium carbonate, the cheapest form, is literally chalk, mined from the ground, and if the supplement just says "calcium" in the list of ingredients, then this is what you are likely to get. It is not a naturally occurring form of calcium, and no foods (either plant or animal) contain it. In addition, it is the most difficult form of calcium to absorb and you need a pretty efficient digestive system in order to manage it. If you have low levels of stomach (hydrochloric) acid, as many women over 40 do, you will struggle to absorb the calcium from a calcium carbonate supplement. One study showed that of a group of post-menopausal women, 40 percent were severely deficient in stomach acid. Those with low levels only absorbed 4 percent of the calcium from calcium carbonate, compared to 45 percent of the calcium from calcium citrate. In fact, calcium citrate is almost 30 percent more absorbable than calcium carbonate.[51]

Two other substances to avoid in calcium supplements are bone meal or dolomite, which may contain high levels of heavy toxic metals such as lead, arsenic, mercury or cadmium. One common calcium supplement, calcium hydroxyapatite, is basically bone meal. It also has relatively low levels (20 percent) of absorption.[52]

How much calcium do you need?

It's not an easy question to answer. Although it has been suggested that women over 45 should take 1,500 milligrams of calcium a day, this is controversial. There is little agreement in the scientific world about the effect of extra calcium in the early postmenopausal years, although it does seem to be effective in reducing bone loss five years or more after menopause.[53]

It is also difficult to know if you are deficient in calcium in the first place. Blood tests for calcium are not particularly helpful because the level of calcium in your blood is no indication of the amount in your bones. In fact, these tests can be misleading, because your body's failsafe mechanism transfers calcium from your bones if levels fall in the blood. Blood calcium concentrations will only be outside normal limits if you are suffering from malnutrition or an overactive thyroid gland. A hair mineral analysis is a better indicator because you can see if there is a high calcium turnover).

In any case, a high calcium intake is not necessarily a good thing. Although you would think that the greater your consumption of calcium, the stronger your bones will be, the reverse could well be true. The irony is that hip fractures occur more frequently in countries such as Scandinavia and The Netherlands, which have a high intake of calcium, and are less common in countries where the average is low.

continued

These findings were backed up by the *American Journal of Clinical Nutrition* in 2001 when it asked, "Why do populations who consume low-calcium diets have fewer fractures than Western societies who consume high-calcium diets?"[54] An example is the Gambia in West Africa, where there is little evidence of osteoporosis despite an average calcium intake of only 300mg a day. The secret may lie in their broadly vegetarian diet. In the Gambia, the average protein intake a day is 40 grams, only 12 grams of which comes from animal sources.[55]

The following table shows that countries that have the highest calcium intake also have the highest rate of hip fractures.

	Animal Protein (g per day)	Calcium Intake (mg per day)	Hip Fractures (100,000 persons)
South Africa	10	196	7
Singapore	25	389	22
Hong Kong	35	356	46
Spain	47	766	42
Great Britain	57	977	118
Denmark	58	960	165
Sweden	59	1104	188
Finland	60	1332	111
USA	72	973	145
New Zealand	78	1217	119

(Source: M Messina et al., *The Simple Soybean and Your Health* [1994], Avery Publishing, New York)

BORON

Boron is another mineral that is being widely studied in relation to osteoporosis. Boron is found naturally in alfalfa, kelp, cabbage and leafy greens, but research conducted by the Department of Agriculture has demonstrated that supplements also have a part to play. Giving post-menopausal women a short course of 3-milligram boron supplements daily resulted in a 44 percent reduction in the amount of calcium excreted in their urine.[56] Boron also helps to activate vitamin D and thereby aid calcium absorption.

Since changes in memory and mental function can be a problem at menopause, it is interesting to note that boron can have positive benefits for the brain as well as the bones. Certainly, short periods of restricted boron intake have been shown to impair brain function and mental performance in healthy men and women.[57]

ZINC

Zinc helps vitamin D to absorb calcium[58] and is also needed for the proper formation of osteoclasts and osteoblasts, the two cells that are essential for renewing bone. Older people with osteoporosis can be deficient in zinc.[59]

IPRIFLAVONE

Ipriflavone is an artificial copy of a soy isoflavone that has been shown to increase bone density in some cases,[60] though not all.[61] More important could be its beneficial effect on bone turnover. Studies show that one of the bone turnover markers in the urine goes down by 29 percent when women take ipriflavone, indicating that bone turnover is reduced. In women taking a placebo this slowing down of bone loss did not happen.[62] More research needs to be done into ipriflavone, especially as one study found that 13 percent of the women taking it had developed a reduction in lymphocytes, the disease fighting white blood cell.

ESSENTIAL FATTY ACIDS

The oils from nuts, seeds and oily fish (the omega 6 and omega 3 essential fatty acids, see page 57) are especially important for your bones. It seems that having good levels of omega 3 fatty acids from oily fish and flax seed can improve both calcium absorption and bone density.[63]

Your supplement plan

To keep your bones healthy before, during and after menopause, try:

• A good multi-vitamin and mineral tablet containing boron
• B complex (50 milligrams of each B vitamin per day, including the amount you get from your multi-vitamin and mineral tablet)
• Vitamin C with bioflavonoids (1,000 milligrams per day)
• A combined magnesium and calcium citrate supplement (with no more than 500 milligrams of calcium citrate per day, including the amount you get from your multi-vitamin and mineral tablet)
• Zinc citrate (15mg a day, including the amount you get from your multi-vitamin and mineral tablet)
• Flax seed oil (1,000mg a day)

Food sources for the bone-friendly nutrients

Calcium – sesame seeds, almonds, canned salmon (including the bones), green leafy vegetables (except spinach), soy, brazil nuts, hazel nuts, dairy products in moderation

Magnesium – nuts, seeds, whole grains, green leafy vegetables

Vitamin C – cauliflower, citrus fruits, berries, potatoes, green leafy vegetables

Zinc – pumpkin seeds, fish, eggs, peas and beans, whole grains

Vitamin D – oily fish, eggs

Boron – cabbage, alfalfa, green vegetables, fruits, nuts, peas and beans

Folic acid – vegetables

Beneficial bacteria – live organic yogurt

Vitamin K – cabbage, alfalfa and green leafy vegetables

Homeopathic remedies

It is usually best to opt for a consultation with a homeopath so that treatment can be tailored to your individual needs. If you want to treat yourself, the main remedies would include calcarea carbonica and calcarea phosphorica.

Treat with respect ...

Vitamin A

This is a vitamin women need to be wary of in connection with menopause and osteoporosis. Taking between 1,500 and 2,000 micrograms of vitamin A (retinol) a day for a long period is known to decrease bone density and increase the risk of hip fractures in women after menopause, although levels of less than 500 micrograms a day do not have this effect. It seems that vitamin A alters the way the body uses calcium and affects bone formation, suppressing osteoblast formation (the cells that build up new bone) and stimulating osteoclast activity (the cells that dissolve bone), so bone is lost.[64] Vitamin A is found in liver, dairy products, fortified margarine and fish oils and it is possible that your bones could be weakened by a diet high in these foods, even if you avoid taking extra vitamin A in the form of health supplements.[65]

However, none of the above applies to carotenes like beta-carotene, found in brightly colored fruit and vegetables such as carrots, sweet potatoes, apricots, green vegetables, pumpkins, apples and peaches. Beta-carotene is a substance that your body converts into vitamin A when you need it, and it does not appear to increase the risk of fractures whether it comes from the diet or is taken as supplements.[66]

So should you avoid vitamin A in animal foods and stick to beta-carotene from fruit and vegetables? No, because vitamin A is a powerful antioxidant, important for the immune system and healthy eyes, preventing poor night vision and dry eyes. My advice would be to carry on eating foods such as oily fish (which is rich in vitamin A) but to eliminate liver. Because vitamin A is stored in the liver, the amount here will be high, a fact acknowledged by the Inuit people who have always avoided the livers of polar bears and seals, knowing that they can fall ill if they eat them. I would also advise caution when choosing supplements. It is better to avoid cod liver oil and to buy supplements where the oil is extracted from the body of the fish instead, because the vitamin A content will be lower.

Another good reason to steer clear of liver is that it is the body's waste-disposal unit. Because it removes pollutants as they pass through body, it often contains a high concentration of toxins.

Lifestyles factors that help to build bone

EXERCISE

Exercise is extremely important in the prevention of osteoporosis. You need to ensure that you are doing some weight-bearing exercise that puts pressure on your bones – take your pick from brisk walking, running, tennis, badminton, stair-climbing and aerobics. Over the years our lifestyles have changed, and we have become more sedentary. We now have washing machines, most of us use the car to go shopping, and many jobs involve sitting behind a computer. We're also busier, but despite that, it's important to make time for exercise and fit it into your schedule. Don't be tempted to put it at the bottom of your to-do list. It is a priority for the prevention of osteoporosis and a wide range of other health conditions.

STRESS

Stress is bad for your bones. The reason for this is that when you are stressed, you produce adrenaline (see page 66) which should really only be brought into play in a life-threatening situation. Unfortunately, many of us live extremely stressful lives and adrenaline is pumped out on a daily basis. As a result, your body believes you are in danger, and puts you on the alert, ready to fight or flee.

There are two issues here. First of all, the adrenal glands are not limitless. They can become exhausted and fail to function properly, which can be very negative in the case of osteoporosis. As we have already seen (page 64), the adrenal glands are able to produce estrogen at menopause, when production from the ovaries starts to fail. If the adrenal glands are worn out, they won't be able to perform this crucial task.

Secondly, when you are stressed, your energy is diverted away from everyday functions such as digestion, which means that you won't be getting the nutrients you need from your food. In the long run that can lead to severe malnutrition, which will undoubtedly affect the health of your bones.

STABLE WEIGHT

Do not lose a lot of weight after middle age unless you are obese or severely overweight as it dramatically increases your chance of a hip fracture. Women who lose more than 10 percent of their weight after the age of 50 can double their risk of a fracture compared to women whose weight remains stable.

Your osteoporosis prevention plan

• It's very important to have your bones monitored regularly, particularly if you are at higher risk of osteoporosis (see page 83).
• If you find that you have osteoporosis, you will need medical advice. However, you should use the natural program in addition to this to make it more effective. Have your bones reassessed regularly to ensure that the medication is working as it should.
• If your bones are fine, or showing only minor signs of bone loss, follow the natural program and have your bones reassessed to ensure that it is working.
• Make sure that you get plenty of weight-bearing exercise to improve bone health.
• Stop smoking. There's no doubt that smoking will weaken your bones.
• If you are on regular medication, such as steroids, make sure you get your bones tested.
• Ensure that you are not underweight, which can reduce protective estrogen levels in the body.
• Make sure that you are eating well.
• Cut caffeine, sugar, alcohol and fizzy drinks out of your diet as much as possible.
• Don't drink tea with meals.
• Avoid eating bran, except in its natural, whole form (see page 97).
• Take a good program of supplements.

CHAPTER 8

Natural Alternatives to HRT

The story so far

An impressive amount of information and research has emerged that has focused on alternative ways of managing menopause, leading to a growing interest in a natural, less medicated approach. Increasing numbers of women have become aware that HRT is the not the wonder-drug it was originally supposed to be and that it does have risks, notably an increased risk of breast cancer and heart disease. At the same time, the rise of the Internet has given women access to medical research previously restricted to doctors and scientists. As women have become more knowledgeable, they have started asking more questions, demanding to know what choices they have in dealing with what is, after all, a natural event in their lives.

I am as convinced as I ever was that hormone replacement therapy should not be the first resort for women at menopause. I am concerned that it is often prescribed as soon as they start to experience symptoms and that many women continue to take it for a period of years. In many cases I feel it is unlikely that all these symptoms are a direct result of menopause, although the changes that occur at this time may certainly exacerbate them and act as a catalyst for existing problems. Our diets, our lifestyles and our lack of essential nutrients may well be exposed by this particular event. For while hot flashes and vaginal dryness may be specific to menopause, other symptoms such as mood swings, painful breasts and water retention are often associated with pre-menstrual problems as well.

As we have seen, once a woman reaches a certain age, it is all too easy to label all her symptoms as "menopausal." Many of these symptoms are less to do with an actual shortage of hormones and much more to do with an imbalance. It is restoring the balance, rather than pumping yourself full of foreign hormones, that alleviates the symptoms of menopause. There are numerous ways to do this. As well as getting our nutrition right we can use natural therapies to combat particular problems and improve our overall health.

Even symptoms that are correctly associated with menopause need more careful consideration than the blanket prescription of HRT, because there is more going on than a drop in hormone levels. We know, for example, that up to 85 percent of Western women experience hot flashes compared to only 14 percent of women in some Asian countries. This is not simply a physiological difference. The interesting thing is that the symptoms of menopause can vary within a culture depending on lifestyle. In China for example, professional, working women experience significantly more menopausal symptoms than women who are farmers living in rural areas.[1]

All this makes it even more important to try different approaches to menopause before resorting to powerful drugs. Any shortcomings in your lifestyle or diet, especially if you are low in essential nutrients, may well become obvious at this time, and simply adjusting your diet can make a world of difference. If this is not enough, natural medicines can do an enormous amount to combat particular problems and improve your overall health. The natural approach has the added benefit of leading to a fuller understanding of the way your body works. Once you have grasped this, it becomes clear that menopause is not a medical condition but a natural event that given the chance, your body should cope with perfectly happily.

Taking responsibility

Because the natural approach is holistic, it is not an easy option. A major difference between the conventional and natural ways of treating menopause is that the natural approach requires a lot more effort. It is certainly easier to pop a pill containing HRT that reduces or removes any symptoms you may have. You can carry on with your current lifestyle and ignore any adverse effects it may have on your health. If you opt for the natural route, however, you will be asked to take responsibility for your health. You will need to monitor the way you live, looking at what you eat, how much you exercise, and how much stress you experience.

Although this requires a long-term commitment, the changes are well worth the effort involved because the benefits extend far beyond menopause. You are not only addressing the menopausal symptoms but also working on preventing or minimizing the diseases associated with aging.

This is important because we live at a time when degenerative diseases have become epidemic. Illnesses such as heart disease, cancer, stroke, diabetes and arthritis are on the increase and very few people in the West now die simply of "old age." If you start to improve your health now, you will be much more likely to prevent problems in the future.

The best therapies for menopause

The therapies I have set out here are those that I have found most helpful in treating symptoms of menopause. Of course, the list is not exhaustive. There are many natural therapies and there is no room to mention them all. Osteopathy and reflexology, for example, can be very helpful. If you have the opportunity, such natural therapies are well worth trying, either alone or in combination with the therapies below. Remember, too, that you can use them in conjunction with conventional medicine. You must also bear in mind, however, that everyone is different, and you may find that some therapies work better for you than others.

NUTRITIONAL THERAPY

Most of us don't realize it but food is, and should be, regarded as a powerful medicine that has a huge impact on the biochemical processes of the body. Nutritional therapy is not just about eating well. It is also about correcting any vitamin or mineral deficiencies. You need to eat a good variety of food and not restrict yourself to a small range, to give yourself the best chance of getting all the nutrients you need. You then need to look at any particular symptoms to see if there are areas that may require supplementation. It's important to remember that supplements are just that – extra – and not a substitute for healthy food. You cannot eat junk food and take nutritional supplements and hope to stay healthy.

You may ask why you need food supplements when many experts say you can get everything you need from a well-balanced diet. Unfortunately, I believe the well-balanced diet is a myth and that in most cases, it is impossible to get all the nutrients you need from food. Part of the problem is that intensive farming methods have depleted the soil of valuable minerals, and if nutrients are lacking in the soil then they are going to be low in the vegetables that are grown from it. For example, the average intake of selenium (a powerful antioxidant) is now only 34 micrograms a day, about half the amount it was 25 years ago.

It is not only the soil that is devoid of nutrients. Much of the food eaten today is so overprocessed that, for example, only one in 10 people receives the RDA (Recommended Daily Allowance) of 15 milligrams for zinc.

Of course it could be argued that HRT is a supplement just as vitamins and minerals are, and that by taking it you are only supplying what your body lacks. There is, however, a major difference between nutritional supplements and HRT. Hormones are chemical compounds produced internally by the body itself. HRT, a powerful drug, contains hormones synthesized – made in a laboratory – from an external source and then introduced into the body. Vitamins and minerals, on the other hand, are obtained from food and in general cannot be produced internally.

Food (or food supplements that provide the same nutrients, albeit in a more concentrated form) gives your body the foundation it needs to build on for good health. From the food you eat and the nutrients that food gives you, your body is able to produce whatever hormones are required. If you are not in good health or your hormones are out of balance, your wisest course is to return to basics and obtain the nutrients you need in the form of food and/or food supplements. By doing so, you will restore your health, allowing your body to produce the correct level of hormones again and get them back in balance.

The vitamins and minerals required to keep your body healthy work in harmony, and most of them depend on each other to act efficiently. So the best way to structure a supplement program is to take a good multi-vitamin and mineral supplement specifically designed for menopause as the foundation of the program. You can then add supplements that relate specifically to any symptoms you have. Take these vitamins and minerals as part of a meal because you want your body to think they are part of your diet and they are better absorbed with food.

When it comes to buying mineral or vitamin supplements, you get what you pay for. Good quality supplements make nutrients more readily available to the body, which is important at menopause. Unfortunately, the digestive system becomes less efficient with age and it is more difficult to process nutrients, so whatever supplements you take need to be readily absorbed. Capsules (preferably vegetable rather than gelatin) are better than tablets. This is because capsules tend to contain only essential nutrients while tablets can include a variety of fillers, binders and bulking agents.

Choosing a supplement is not always straightforward, and it is important to read the label. When buying a mineral supplement like calcium, for example, look for the words citrate, ascorbate or polynicotinate, all of which are more easily absorbed by the body. "Chelated" (pronounced "keylated") minerals are also good. This process makes minerals more digestible because they are "hooked" onto an amino acid, allowing three to 10 times greater assimilation than a non-chelated variety.

Types of calcium to avoid include those described as chlorides, sulphates, carbonates or oxides, which are less easily assimilated and may pass through the body. Be aware of what the label doesn't say, too. If it simply lists calcium as an active ingredient, it is likely to be calcium carbonate, a cheaper supplement that is difficult to absorb.

> Please remember, everyone should consult with a pharmacist or healthcare practitioner to make sure that vitamins or supplements do not interfere with prescribed medications.

HERBS

As with food supplements, herbs can be used to get yourself back into good health so that your body can balance your hormones, heal itself and help to prevent illness and disease from getting a hold. Herbal medicine is the oldest

---

Put your supplements to the test

If you are already taking supplements and want to know how well they are being absorbed, do the following test:
• Place the supplement in a glass of warm vinegar (this roughly represents the conditions found in your digestive tract).
• Leave it for 30 minutes, stirring every few minutes.
• If the supplement does not dissolve after half an hour, then, as the critics say, "you are paying an awful lot for nutritious urine." In other words, the nutrients are probably leaving your body in much the same form as they entered! My recommendation is to buy another brand.

---

form of medicine, and herbs have been used for healing in every single culture since the beginning of civilization. Wise women have always played a central role in human society and knowledge about herbs was passed on from one generation to the next.

Herbs are in fact the foundation of numerous pharmaceutical drugs. Aspirin is based on an extract of willow, originally used for pain relief by Native Americans. Up to 70 percent of drugs in use today have their origins in plants. But Western pharmaceutical practice uses the active ingredient of the plant or herb in a pure form of a determined strength and quantity as the basis for the drug. When a plant or herb is used in its whole form, as in herbal medicine, the side-effects are absent or minimal. In traditional times, the foxglove plant (*Digitalis purpurea*), for example, was used for heart problems. In modern times, scientists have been able to isolate the main active ingredient of the foxglove (digoxin). However, by using only the active ingredient in a drug form, there is a real risk of side-effects. By using the whole plant, the active ingredient interacts with all the other constituents of the plant, which actually include "buffer" ingredients that counteract the side-effects. Herbalists believe this is the proper way to use the healing powers of herbs and plants.

The best way to use herbs is to choose those that have a balancing effect on your hormones without directly supplying one hormone or another. These balancing agents are called adaptogens. Adaptogenic herbs allow the body to restore itself naturally without causing an imbalance in any hormone or body system. These herbs tone and strengthen the whole of the reproductive system. Examples are chasteberry (*Agnus castus*) and black cohosh. Below I have given a guide to the general use of these and other herbs at menopause. If you have specific symptoms such as fibroids, for instance, it would be worth consulting a good herbalist or a health professional with experience in using herbs because some can have a direct hormone-like action and are used in specific conditions, but are best avoided for others.

For general use, it is better to have a number of herbs mixed together. Some herbs work better for some women than others, so if you take an appropriate "menopause" mix you can be sure of having a good balance.

The easiest and most effective way of taking herbs is in tincture form (approximately 1 teaspoon, three times daily in a little water). Try to get tinctures made from organically grown herbs. In liquid form, the herbs are already dissolved and hence they are available faster and their action is quicker. If you find that you don't like the taste of herbs in liquid form or find it more convenient to use capsules, then good "menopause" mixes of powdered herbs are available in vegetable capsules.

Herbs are not like drugs. If drugs are stopped, the symptoms can return and you are back where you started. The herbs stop the symptoms, but they also address the cause at the same time, so the symptoms are being alleviated because the body is becoming more balanced.

HOMEOPATHY

The word "homeopathy" comes from the Greek *omio,* meaning "same" and *pathos* meaning "suffering." It is a treatment of using like with like, based on a system for treating a disease based on administering minute closes of a substance that in larger does produces symptoms in a healthy person. Homeopathy was founded by Samuel Hahnemann, a German doctor, and is an extremely safe form of medicine which works on the principle of helping the body to fight its own battles. The remedy given contains only the most minute quantities of a substance. It is in direct contrast to conventional medicine, which treats symptoms by trying to create the opposite effect to that from which the person is suffering. If a person is feeling very stressed, anxious and has palpitations, for instance, a homeopathic remedy could be given that in a healthy person would actually create that same set of symptoms, thereby encouraging the body's own healing mechanisms. Modern conventional medicine, on the other hand, would prescribe drugs such as tranquilizers and beta blockers to create calmness.

In homeopathy, different women may be prescribed different remedies for the same problem. Homeopaths take a very detailed history and not only look at the symptoms the person is suffering from now but also find out likes and dislikes, whether they are a hot or cold person, their sleeping patterns, emotional factors and much more. The remedy prescribed is then called a "constitutional remedy" and is individual to that person.

The remedies listed below are "symptomatic," but if your symptoms have shown no sign of improvement for some time, it would be better to seek help from a qualified homeopath who will be able to treat you constitutionally.

Several homeopathic remedies are recommended for menopause and they can be chosen depending on the kind and severity of symptoms you are experiencing. These remedies are to be taken every twelve hours for up to seven days at a potency of 30x. (30x is a measure of the concentration of a remedy. The higher the number, the more potent the remedy.)

• Sepia is one of the main remedies for menopause. It is useful for heavy periods, hot flashes, headaches and also if you are easily depressed and irritable.
• Lachesis is for flooding during periods, irritability, forgetfulness, hot flashes and a headache on waking.
• Pulsatilla is especially suited to those with fair hair and who cry easily.
• Kali carb is useful if the symptoms are worse in the middle of the night and also where there is loss of appetite.
• Graphites is beneficial for those women who have scanty periods, weight gain and hot flashes.
• Sanguinaria is useful for tender breasts and heavy periods.
• Conium is helpful where there is a lack of sex drive.

AROMATHERAPY

Aromatherapy is the use of essential oils, and has been popular for centuries. Egyptians used frankincense for embalming and Cleopatra was reputed to have seduced Mark Antony by wearing jasmine oil. Hippocrates, the father of medicine, stated that "the way to good health is to take an aromatic bath and fragrant massage every day." During the two world wars, clove, thyme and chamomile oils were used as substitutes for scarce disinfectants.

The term "aromatherapy" was used in the 1930s by the French chemist René Gatefosse. While working in a laboratory, he burned his hand and plunged it into a nearby bowl of lavender oil. The burn healed quickly with little scarring. Impressed by this, he began to investigate the medicinal powers of pure essential oils. Essential oils are found in the stems, flowers, leaves, bark, seeds or peel of aromatic plants. Once extracted, these become more concentrated and potent. Each essential oil has its own specific properties and works on two levels: through our sense of smell and by being absorbed into the bloodstream via the skin and lungs, where it has a therapeutic effect on organs, glands and tissue. The oils are volatile, so must be kept in dark glass bottles out of the sun and at a cool temperature. If the essential oil is to come into contact with your skin it must be blended in a carrier oil, such as almond oil (exceptions are lavender oil and tea tree oil) or diluted in water. Drops of essential oil can be used directly in the bath.

The most suitable oils for menopause are chamomile, geranium, rose, jasmine, neroli, ylang-ylang, bergamot, sandalwood and clary sage. There are a number of ways of using them.

Massage

The aim of massage is to target problem areas by stroking, pressing and kneading each area of the body in turn to relieve pain, relax, stimulate and tone it. Massage also stimulates the circulation and assists the lymphatic system (which runs parallel to the circulatory system), improving the elimination of toxic waste from the body. Oils are frequently used to make the massage more comfortable and effective, and adding pure essential oils to the mix means that you can benefit from their healing power too. It is a good idea to take a bath or shower before a massage so that the oil is better absorbed. If you want to massage a partner, or try self-massage, use five drops of essential oil to 2 teaspoons of carrier oil. If you have sensitive skin, you can use jojoba oil as a carrier, but never use aromatherapy oils or give a massage on broken or infected skin.

Bath or shower

Add five drops of essential oil to the water just before you step into the bath so that the oil is strong. The room should be warm, but the water shouldn't be too hot or the oil will disperse quickly. Soak for 10 to 15 minutes and inhale the steam as you do so. If you prefer to take a shower, stay under the spray and massage yourself with the oil using a mitt or sponge. Use five drops of essential oil in 2 teaspoons of carrier oil. You can also take advantage of aromatherapy by using a footbath. Put four drops of essential oil in a bowl of warm water and soak your feet for 15 to 20 minutes.

Steam inhalation

Fill a basin with hot water, add two to three drops of essential oil and lean over it, covering your head with a towel so that none of the aromatic steam escapes. Breathe deeply for five minutes, keeping your eyes closed.

Other ways to inhale include:

• placing a few drops on a tissue or pillow
• adding a few drops to a bowl of water near a radiator, so the oil vaporizes

- adding eight drops of oil to ¹¹⁄₄₂ pint of water to use as a room spray
- using scented light bulb rings, essential oil burners and steam vaporizers

Acupuncture

This ancient Chinese system of medicine dates back some 2,000 years and can be particularly useful for treating menopausal symptoms. It is based on the concept of Qi, or chi (pronounced "chee"), which is the body's energy. An acupuncturist aims to balance the flow of Qi along pathways called meridians. By inserting fine needles into the meridians, the body's own healing response can be stimulated.

Acupuncture can be used with the other natural medicine therapies to correct hormone and energy imbalances during menopause. This is obviously not a self-help system, so you need to see a qualified acupuncturist.

Natural ways to treat menopausal symptoms

You might suffer from a single menopausal symptom or several together, or all of them at different times. But it is pretty safe to say that you would not be reading this book if you didn't have any of them at all.

In response to the many letters I have received from readers, and to the questions asked in the clinic and at seminars, I have updated and expanded the information to include the latest findings together with some extra sections, set out here in alphabetical order:

Aching joints
Anxiety and irritability
Breast tenderness
Constipation
Depression
Fatigue/lack of energy
Hair loss
Headaches and migraines
Heavy periods
Hot flashes and night sweats
Lack of libido
Memory/concentration
Painful periods
Skin problems
Sleep problems
Stress incontinence

Vaginal dryness
Water retention

To make the information fully comprehensive, I have tried to cover as wide a range of menopausal symptoms as possible and provide specific detailed advice, so you will have the knowledge you need to treat them naturally.

ACHING JOINTS

Many women I see complain of stiffness and painful joints, which frequently become a problem at menopause. If you are affected, my first recommendation is to increase your intake of essential fatty acids (EFAs) contained in nuts, seeds, oily fish and some vegetables. These encourage the body to produce "good" prostaglandins, the hormone-like substances that help to decrease inflammation in the joints. Research has shown that eating just one portion of oily fish a day can have a dramatic effect on rheumatoid arthritis.[2] At the same time as stepping up your consumption of EFAs, it is wise to eliminate or cut down on dairy foods and red meat for a while because they contribute to the production of one of the "bad" prostaglandins that can increase inflammation and pain in the joints.

Falling estrogen levels can also contribute to painful joints, so phytoestrogens in the form of soy, chickpeas, lentils and so on should be a regular part of your diet. Aching and painful joints can also be a sign of food allergy, so check the other symptoms on page 186 to see whether this could be the culprit.

Nutritional therapy

As the essential fatty acids are so vital for your joints it is worth adding them in as supplements. As we eat these oils (Omega 3 and Omega 6) our bodies make them more and more complex. The Omega 6 oils (from sunflower, sesame, walnuts, flax seed and soy) are converted to gamma-linolenic (GLA) which is found in evening primrose oil. The Omega 3 oils (from oily fish, flax seed, walnuts, soy, pumpkin and green leafy vegetables) are converted to eicospentaenoc acid (EPA) which is found directly in oily fish. Some people have problems converting these oils into GLA and EPA so if you are suffering from aching and painful joints, get them in supplement form where the conversion has already taken place – that is, in the form of GLA and EPA.

The sulphur MSM (methyl sulphonyl methane) occurs naturally in food. It helps to maintain healthy connective tissue, keeping the joints flexible and reducing pain. So it is a useful supplement to take if you are getting joint pains, together with glucosamine sulphate, which stimulates the production of substances needed for the joints to mend and move more easily. Glucosamine has been used in a number of clinical trials on osteoarthritis, where it has been found to relieve joint pain and improve mobility.[3]

Bromelain is an enzyme contained in pineapples which has anti-inflammatory properties. It helps to decrease the level of "bad" prostaglandins that cause pain and inflammation and increase the "good" prostaglandins, which do the opposite.[4]

Take:
Multi-vitamin and mineral supplement designed for menopause
GLA (150mg)
EPA (300mg)
Glucosamine sulphate (1,000mg)
MSM (2,000-3,000mg)
Bromelain (500mg, 3 times a day between meals)

Note:
Each nutrient represents the total intake for one day, so look at the contents of your multi-vitamin and mineral supplement and just add in any extras to the recommended amounts.

Herbs
One of the most useful herbs for relieving painful joints is devil's claw, which seems to reduce both inflammation and pain. Boswellic acid is also helpful for aching joints. It appears to improve the blood supply to the joints even if they have been damaged by arthritis.

Aromatherapy
Oils like lavender, chamomile, bergamot and rose can be very helpful. One of the easiest ways to use them is to add a few drops to a relaxing bath. Lavender is useful if the joints are very painful, and juniper is excellent for swelling.

ANXIETY AND IRRITABILITY
Make sure that you keep your blood sugar level in balance. This is explained on page 67. It is important that you eliminate "stimulants" such as alcohol, tea, coffee and sugar which give a quick rise in blood sugar followed by a drop. As your blood sugar levels drop, your body will release adrenaline to try to correct this imbalance. Adrenaline is the hormone that is also released when you are under stress, so you can feel those same feelings of anxiety and tension even when there is no external stress at all. Eat little and often for the same reason. If you go more than three hours without food adrenaline will be released into the system again.

Nutritional therapy

Several minerals and vitamins can help to reduce stress. Magnesium, for example, is often called "nature's tranquilizer," so it is worth taking as a supplement. The B vitamins are also well known for their ability to help with stress, so these should be included too.

Take:
Multi-vitamin and mineral supplements designed for menopause
Magnesium (300mg)
Vitamin B complex (containing 50mg of each B vitamin)

Note:
Each nutrient represents the total intake for one day, so look at the contents of your multi-vitamin and mineral supplement and just add in any extras to the recommended amounts.

Herbs

In herbal medicine, herbs that help us to feel calm are called "nervines." They act on the nervous system to relieve anxiety, tension and irritability and induce calm. One of the best-known herbs for anxiety and tension is valerian. It is often effective when combined with skullcap, which also relaxes the nervous system. Skullcap is also useful for pre-menstrual syndrome (PMS) and because this is closely associated with irritability, it is a good herb to choose at menopause.

Another herbal remedy that helps with both pre-menstrual and menopausal tension is *Agnus castus*. Women suffering from PMS who often feel worse in the years leading up to menopause may find it especially beneficial because *Agnus castus* is the most important herb in the treatment of PMS. The latest research confirming its benefits was reported in the *British Medical Journal* in 2001.[5] It stated that more than half the women who had been taking *Agnus castus* reported a 50 percent or greater improvement in their symptoms, an effect that was experienced in just three cycles. The research concluded that "*Agnus castus* is a well tolerated and effective treatment for pre-menstrual syndrome, the effects being confirmed by physicians and patients alike. The effects are detected in most main symptoms of the syndrome."

The third option for treating anxiety and tension is ginseng. Panax (Korean or Chinese) ginseng is often used as a tonic because it improves the function of the adrenal glands. Studies have shown that the use of panax ginseng can help people withstand the effects of many different stressful situations and increases mental alertness; it can also boost vitality and physical performance. Siberian ginseng also helps to combat stress but has a more subtle effect than panax ginseng and can be used over a longer period of time. Both types of ginseng are classed as adaptogens because they have a normalizing, balancing effect on the body.

Aromatherapy

Clary sage is wonderful for lifting your mood and seems to be particularly effective blended with geranium. Put 7 drops of clary sage and 7 drops of geranium in a carrier oil. Use in your bath or as a massage.

BREAST TENDERNESS

Up to 70 percent of women have fibrocystic breasts – tender swollen breasts and swollen lumps that fluctuate with the menstrual cycle and may become more obvious and painful in the very early stages of menopause. Excess estrogen may be the cause of this rather frightening condition, which is not, however, thought to have any link to breast cancer. Avoid drinks that contain methylxanthines (coffee, tea, chocolate, cola and even decaffeinated coffee) as these have been shown to cause breast lumps.[6]

We are exposed to excess hormones (xenoestrogens) from both the plastics and pesticide industries, so try to reduce your exposure by choosing organic foods where possible.

Phytoestrogens, those weak, naturally occurring estrogens (see page 48), can help to keep any excesses of estrogen in check and may explain why the majority of Asian women do not experience breast discomfort as we do. Phytoestrogens are effectively "plant" estrogens, and they are found in foods such as soy, chickpeas and lentils. Include them all in your diet as often as you can.

The belief that sore breasts can be caused by surplus estrogen helps to explain findings that there is a link between fibrocystic breast disease and constipation. It has been suggested that certain microorganisms in bowel matter are capable of recycling estrogen that would otherwise be excreted, and so failing to eliminate waste and toxic products from the body is literally storing up trouble. One research paper in *The Lancet* showed that women who had fewer than three bowel movements per week had a 4.5 times greater chance of having breast problems than women who had a bowel movement at least once a day.[7] Another study found that women who ate a vegetarian diet excreted three times more "old" estrogens than women who ate meat, so that these hormones were eliminated from their system and no longer recycled. It seems that dietary fiber from grains and vegetables reduces estrogen levels by preventing constipation and also prevents estrogens in the bile from being reabsorbed back into the blood. However, adding wheat bran is not the ideal solution as this can irritate the bowel and may prevent the uptake of essential nutrients in the digestive tract. The answer is to eat more whole foods.

A diet high in saturated fats is known to stimulate the overproduction of estrogen, so a low-fat diet may help to reduce breast tenderness and pain.[8] But although avoiding all animal products, except fish, could help, don't fall into the trap of thinking that a "no-fat" diet would be even better. Essential fats (see page 55) are beneficial, so try to increase your intake of oily fish, nuts and seeds.

Nutritional therapy

You can boost your consumption of essential fats by taking a supplement of fish oil, flax seed oil or evening primrose oil. Vitamin E also helps to relieve breast pain. Adding in a supplement containing beneficial bacteria (a probiotic such as *Lactobacillus acidophilus*) can also help because it lowers the level of the enzymes that recycle estrogen in the body, so more is excreted. Another way to encourage the elimination of excess estrogen is to take a B complex supplement. This is because a deficiency of B vitamins can prevent the liver from deactivating waste estrogen.

Take:
Multi-vitamin and mineral supplement designed for menopause
Vitamin E (400–1,000iu)
Flax seed oil (1,000mg)
Probiotic (morning and night)
Vitamin B complex (50mg twice a day)

Note:
Each nutrient represents the total intake for one day, so look at the contents of your multi-vitamin and mineral supplement and just add in any extras to the recommended amounts.

Herbs

Because lumpy or tender breasts may be a sign that estrogen is not being processed efficiently by the liver, some beneficial herbs for the liver may help to boost this process.

Dandelion helps to cleanse the liver, the major organ of detoxification which also gets rid of accumulated "old" female hormones. If the liver is functioning effectively, this prevents excess estrogen from building up and increasing the risk of breast growth and cell changes.

Milk thistle is also an excellent herb for the liver and several studies have shown that its use can result in an increase in new liver cells to replace old damaged ones.[9] Silymarin is the collective name for the substances found in milk thistle which have this beneficial effect.

Agnus castus can be used for breast tenderness because of its ability to normalize the female hormones.[10] Using this herb can help to correct any imbalances of excess estrogen.

CONSTIPATION

It is essential to keep your bowels working properly because their function is to get rid of everything your body doesn't want or need, and that includes "old" hormones, especially estrogen. If you do not dispose of toxins efficiently, there is a risk that these may be re-absorbed. So make sure you help your digestive system work smoothly by eating a good supply of fruits and vegetables and drinking plenty of water.

Improving your diet in this way is much better than relying on laxatives. Most laxatives work by stimulating or increasing the number of bowel movements you have, or by encouraging a softer or bulkier stool. Unfortunately they do not address the cause of the problem, such as lack of fiber, and people can become dependent on them. The more these laxatives are used, the less the body has to do for itself, and ultimately it can mean that the bowel loses its tone and muscle action. The end result is that the person cannot do without the laxatives.

As awareness of these problems has grown, increasing the amount of fiber in the diet has become popular. Unfortunately, the focus has been on adding bran to increase the fiber content of a poor and over-refined diet, which completely misses the point. Bran is a refined food too, because it is extracted from the grains of cereal plants. It also contains phytates, which mop up vital nutrients such as zinc and magnesium, making it harder for your body to absorb them. These phytates also interfere with the uptake of calcium, which is essential for the health of your bones during menopause. So it makes much more sense to take bran in the form that nature intended by eating the grains in their whole state.

If you want a simple remedy for constipation, try flax seed rather than bran – they are far more effective. Simply soak a tablespoon of whole flax seed in water for about 20 minutes and swallow them whole, at breakfast time. It is important to realize that there is a difference between using flax seed to improve the action of your bowels and taking it for its nutrient value. Normally you should grind the seeds so your body can absorb the nutrients. (Flax seed is rich in phytestrogens and it is estimated that one tablespoon of flax seed is equivalent to one portion of soy.) Otherwise, the seeds can pass out in the same form they went in!

Nutritional therapy

Take:

Multi-vitamin and mineral supplement designed for menopause

Vitamin C (3,000mg increasing by 500mg daily until your stools are soft and comfortable)

Flax seed oil capsules (1,000mg twice a day)

Note:

Each nutrient represents the total intake for one day, so look at the contents of your multi-vitamin and mineral supplement and just add in any extras to the recommended amounts.

Herbs

Herbs work in two ways to correct constipation. First, they help to create a healthy and frequent bowel movement, and second, they tone the bowel so it regains its natural function. Among the most helpful herbs are butternut, blue flag and physillium. Ready-made remedies include capsules that contain a number of gentle bowel-toning herbs, and capsules or powders designed to cleanse the bowel and detoxify the colon.

DEPRESSION

For some women, the psychological symptoms of menopause are a bigger problem than the physical ones such as hot flashes. They can feel very emotional, crying for no particular reason or feeling very weepy when watching a film that would not have made them feel that way before. Some women just feel very sad, while others are actually depressed.

It is vital to make sure that your blood sugar is balanced to avoid surges of the stress hormone, adrenaline. This can be done by eating little and often, and avoiding caffeine and sugar completely for a couple of months. After that, you can reintroduce them as an occasional treat.

Nutritional therapy

Adding a B-complex supplement helps to counteract depression. The B vitamins are known as the "stress" vitamins and B6 is especially important because it is needed to make serotonin, the "antidepressant" brain chemical. You should also include magnesium, which is a natural tranquilizer, and some essential fatty acids, such as flax seed oil capsules, which are important for healthy brain function.

Take:
Multi-vitamin and mineral supplement containing boron
Vitamin B complex (50mg of most of the B vitamins)
Flax seed oil (1,000mg)
Magnesium (200mg)

Note:
Each nutrient represents the total intake for one day, so look at the contents of your multi-vitamin and mineral supplement and just add in any extras to the recommended amounts.

Herbs

Although St. John's wort (*Hypericum perforatum*) has been used for centuries as a natural antidepressant, interest in it has soared over the past five years. The claims made for it were substantiated in 1996, when a review of 23 studies published in the *British Medical Journal* showed that it is an effective treatment for depression, sleep problems and anxiety.[11] It is interesting to note that a study published in the *Journal of the American Medical Association* in 2002 reported that St. John's wort was no more effective than a placebo in treating moderate to severe depression. However, keep in mind that the subjects of this study had moderate to severe depression and St. John's wort is known to be beneficial only for mild to moderate depression, so a negative result is not surprising. St. John's wort is still considered to be beneficial for mild depression. Another interesting point not widely publicized is that the standard antidepressant used in the trial was also found to be less effective than a placebo.

St. John's wort grows freely in Europe, Asia and America and is often classed as a weed. It has yellow flowers with small red dots on the petals which contain hypericin, a compound that scientists believe can help to lift depression. It is thought to work by increasing levels of the feel-good brain chemicals, serotonin, dopamine and noradrenaline, in the same way as SSRI (selective serotonin reuptake inhibitor) antidepressants such as Prozac.

One study that compared St. John's wort with the antidepressant Imipramine found that it was "therapeutically equivalent" to Imipramine – in other words, it worked as well as the antidepressant.[12] Interestingly, it was better tolerated than the drug. Adverse side-effects were reported in 39 percent of the participants taking St. John's wort compared to 63 percent of those taking Imipramine. What's more, only 3 percent of the participants withdrew because of problems with St. John's wort compared to 16 percent of those taking Imipramine.

This means that the plant is effectively working in the same way as a drug, but with fewer side-effects. That doesn't mean that there are none at all. One that sometimes occurs, especially in fair-skinned people, is increased sensitivity to sunlight. This means that people who take St. John's wort have an increased risk of burning when exposed to the sun, which can be particularly problematic if it is taken at high doses for long periods of time. Fortunately the sensitivity ends when you stop taking the herb.

If you are already taking any medication, such as antidepressants, you need to speak to your doctor before starting St. John's wort. It has been suggested that it can stop the contraceptive pill from working properly and there are concerns about interactions with other drugs, such as those for heart problems, blood clots, epilepsy, migraines and also drugs taken after organ transplants and for HIV treatment.

Aromatherapy

Essential oils can be very useful for depression, whether blended and used in a massage or added to a bath. Lavender is calming and relaxing, bergamot, chamomile and rose help to reduce depression and irritability, while clary sage, sandalwood and ylang-ylang are sedative and antidepressant.

FATIGUE/LACK OF ENERGY

First check that your iron and thyroid levels are correct. Your doctor can do this. If the levels are all right, then again look at your blood sugar balance. Are you having regular cups of tea and coffee during the day that is actually making you feel more tired? Do you need another one to keep yourself going? Are you tired because you are not sleeping well as a result of night sweats, or because of too much tea or coffee? A patient of mine went to her doctor because she was lacking in energy all through the day, he told her she had TATT, Tired All The Time! She knew that, of course; what she wanted to know was why, and what could she do about it?

Nutritional therapy

If your iron and thyroid checks are fine, then try supplementing with co-enzyme Q10, which has been shown to increase energy production in our cells. Co-enzyme Q10 is a substance that is present in all human tissues and organs. It is a vital catalyst in the provision of energy for all human cells. The consequence of a deficiency of co-enzyme is a reduction in energy and a slowing down of life-giving processes. A good balanced diet should contain all the Q10 you need, but unfortunately ability to produce Q10 from food decreases with age. As a result, you may need to take a supplement.

Take:
Multi-vitamin and mineral supplement designed for menopause
Co-enzyme Q10 (50-100mg)
Vitamin E (400iu)
Vitamin B complex (100mg of each B vitamin)

Note:
Each nutrient represents the total intake for one day, so look at the contents of your multi-vitamin and mineral supplement and just add in any extras to the recommended amounts.

Herbs

Panax and Siberian ginseng can help boost your energy and vitality. Although it is sometimes necessary for us to keep our energy levels going because we have something to finish or we just haven't time to rest, it is not good to do this with stimulants such as tea or coffee. It creates a vicious circle of needing something more often. The same thing can actually happen with some herbs, too. It is all right to use the ginseng to help increase your energy levels but you also need to look at your overall nutrition and health.

HAIR LOSS

At menopause, some women find that their hair becomes much thinner than it used to be. It may become sparse all over, or just on top of the head. Some women start to lose body hair while others discover that hair is starting to grow, but unfortunately where it is unwanted, on the face.

Shedding up to 100 hairs a day is considered normal so it is worth checking your hairbrush if you are concerned. If you lose more hair than this, or you notice an increase in the rate at which you are losing hair, or you become aware that your hair is noticeably thinner, see your doctor to rule out problems such as anemia (low hemoglobin levels), low iron (ferritin) stores and thyroid disease. Looking at what has been happening in your life over the past few months can provide a clue if there is no obvious medical cause, because extreme hair loss can be triggered by stress.

If your hair is thinning mainly on the top or you are noticing growth of facial hair, this can be due to a change in the balance of hormones. As estrogen declines at menopause, testosterone (the "male" hormone) can become more dominant. You don't necessarily have more testosterone, it just seems like more to your body because the ratio of estrogen to testosterone has changed, which means that you can get symptoms of male pattern baldness or other male characteristics such as facial hair and acne.

But if you are under a lot of stress or have blood sugar swings, both of which release adrenaline, that can increase testosterone levels. Adrenaline creates cholesterol which in turn can produce more testosterone. Including more phytoestrogens in your diet in the form of soy, chickpeas, kidney beans and so on will help to balance excess male hormone.

Surprisingly, hair loss is also a recognized side-effect of taking HRT. It can go either way. Some women who take HRT find that their hair falls out in handfuls while others find that it improves the quality of their hair.

In many cases, of course, hormones have little to do with it and changes in the quantity and quality of your hair are simply a reflection of your general health. Your hair is an extension of your skin, your connective tissue, and needs to be nourished in the same way. Dry hair and soft or brittle nails can be the first signs that your health is not 100 percent. Many women who correct long-term vitamin and mineral deficiencies tell me that not only has their health benefited but also that they have been able to grow their nails for the first time in years.

Hair follicles need energy to grow, so don't skip meals, especially breakfast, because energy levels are lowest in the morning. It is important to eat little and often. Make sure you are eating enough good-quality protein (vegetable and fish), because this is essential for hair growth, and check that your intake of minerals is sufficient. Lack of essential fatty acids (EFAs) is frequently a culprit because so many women follow "no-fat" and "low-fat" diets. To boost your intake of EFAs, eat plenty of oily fish, nuts and seeds, and take a supplement of flax seed oil for about three months.

If your hair is coming out in patches and creating bald spots on your scalp you probably need to see a specialist, because this type of hair loss is not related to menopause. You could consult a trichologist (hair specialist).

Nutritional therapy

One of the main deficiencies linked to hair loss is zinc, so it is worth taking this in supplement form. Vitamins can also contribute to a good head of hair. Vitamin C is important for all connective tissue and vitamin E is thought to play a part in reducing male hormone levels in women.

Take:
Multi-vitamin and mineral supplement designed for menopause
Zinc citrate (50mg)
Vitamin E (600iu)
Vitamin C (1,000mg)

Flax seed oil (1,000mg)
B complex, if stress could be a factor (50mg of most of the B vitamins)

Note:
Each nutrient represents the total intake for one day, so look at the contents of your multi-vitamin and mineral supplement and just add in any extras to the recommended amounts.

Herbs

One of the most effective herbs for hair loss is horsetail, which is a natural silica. Silica forms part of all connective tissue cells, including hair, skin and nails. If stress is a major factor for you, add Siberian ginseng to nourish the adrenal glands.

A herbal rinse containing rosemary can also help to strengthen the hair. Use 1 ounce to 1 pint of water after shampooing.

HEADACHES AND MIGRAINES

There is a difference between a headache and a migraine headache. Headaches are painful but are not usually accompanied by other symptoms; they can be caused by tension or bad posture from sitting in one position for too long. These can be relieved with a hot bath with essential oils or an aromatherapy massage. Good oils to use are melissa and lavender. Lavender, as an essential oil, can be rubbed into the temples directly on to the skin without first being put in a carrier oil.

Migraine headaches, however, usually follow a pattern of symptoms and these can be different for different people depending on the type of migraine they get. Some sufferers experience warning symptoms (aura) before the pain starts, and these can include blurring and changes in vision, yawning and fatigue, and numbness on one side of the body. The pain itself is usually accompanied by nausea and sometimes vomiting. Scientists now seem agreed that migraines are connected with changes in blood vessels, where the vessels first contract and then dilate, causing the pain. Migraines can be one of the side-effects of HRT and can be so debilitating that women have to stop taking it.

Food allergies are a major cause of migraine headaches, and this should be the first thing you look at. Foods containing tyramine, nitrite, monosodium glutamate or alcohol can all be possible suspects. This would include chocolate, cheese and cocoa. Try to work out whether the migraines are triggered by something you eat or drink by following the recommendations on food allergies on page 186.

Some women get a migraine that is linked to the beginning of their period and as they get to menopause, these migraines stop. Other women start to get migraines at menopause that they didn't have before. If you have eliminated any food triggers, then it is likely your migraines are hormonal.

The liver is the organ of detoxification and gets rid of your "old" hormones. If your liver is not functioning properly then these "old" hormones can build up like toxins, resulting in a migraine. The same build-up can cause nausea and vomiting without the pain.

If you are reacting to certain foods, these will also seem like toxins to your body, so again a migraine and nausea can follow when you eat them.

Nutritional therapy

Take:
Multivitamin and mineral supplement designed for menopause
Quercetin (300mg three times a day)
Vitamin C (1,000mg twice a day)
Vitamin E (300iu)
Flax seed oil (1,000mg a day)

Note:
Each nutrient represents the total intake for one day, so look at the contents of your multivitamin and mineral supplement and just add in any extras to the recommended amounts.

Herbs

Feverfew has received a lot of attention as an "anti-migraine" herb, and a study at the London Migraine Clinic, reported in the *British Medical Journal*, showed it could produce remarkable results.[13] However, it is really designed to prevent migraine, not to treat it, and should be taken daily rather than at the time of an attack.

Herbs that have a direct effect on the liver, such as dandelion and milk thistle, can also be very effective in eliminating migraines. Both can help to cleanse it while milk thistle also has the ability to stimulate the production of new liver cells.

Aromatherapy

If your problem is headache rather than migraine, try aromatherapy oils, either in a warm bath or as massage. Good oils to choose are melissa and lavender. Lavender is especially useful as it can be rubbed into the temples directly, without being mixed with a carrier oil.

HEAVY PERIODS (MENORRHAGIA)

You may just have heavy periods. But excessive bleeding could be a symptom of something else that should be investigated. There are a number of conditions that cause heavy bleeding, including fibroids (benign, harmless growths), endometriosis (the uterine lining growing in places other than the uterus, an

Seven-day liver spring-clean

Because the liver is the body's waste-disposal unit, it needs to be working efficiently for you to eliminate toxins and waste products properly. This is especially true at menopause when it is clearing out our "old" hormones. To improve it, try this very gentle detox regime.

Days 1-2 Cut out tea, coffee and alcohol to prepare your body for the cleanse.

Days 3-7 First thing in the morning, before you eat, drink this liver flush to help your body get rid of toxins and give you a spring-cleaning. In a blender mix:

8 fluid ounces of freshly squeezed lemon juice. (If you can't drink that much, use organic apple juice instead with a squeeze of lemon, or sip apple juice to remove any aftertaste.)
8 fluid ounces of spring or mineral water
1 clove of fresh garlic
1 tablespoon of extra virgin olive oil
1¼₄ inch of fresh ginger root

Blend to a smooth liquid and drink slowly. Fifteen minutes later, drink a cup of hot peppermint tea. Eat normally for the rest of the day (you must eat well to keep your blood sugar up) but keep your meals very simple so that your body has the chance to eliminate toxins. Eat plenty of fresh fruit and vegetables, salads, stir-fried vegetables, vegetable soups, brown rice and oatmeal. You may have headaches or flu-like symptoms for the first couple of days, but don't worry – these are an indication that you are detoxifying. You can repeat this program every couple of months if you feel that you benefit from it.

infection (pelvic inflammatory disease), and uterine or cervical cancer. Use of the coil (IUD) for contraception can also be responsible. The cause of the heavy bleeding needs to be checked out first by a doctor.

Fibroids are non-cancerous growths that grow in or on the walls of the uterus and are very common as we get older. It is thought that their growth is caused by an excess of estrogen, so it follows that as we get to menopause the fibroids actually shrink and become less troublesome. They are usually symptomless except for causing heavy periods, and seem to be linked to a later menopause. They can be removed surgically and often a hysterectomy is advised. As fibroids are non-cancerous, it makes sense to try natural therapies first to pre-empt the need for what is really major surgery.

The major factor found in both heavy bleeding and period pains (see page 139) is the increased production of series 2 prostaglandins. This increase seems to be caused by an increase in arachidonic acid. Arachidonic acid is found predominantly in meat and dairy foods, so by reducing these two foods together with taking some essential fatty acids (such as flax seed oil), it is possible to control heavy bleeding and period pains.

Nutritional therapy

If you are bleeding very heavily you may run the risk of becoming anemic. Take some extra iron but not in the form of ferrous sulphate. This is an inorganic mineral, of which only 2-10 percent is actually absorbed – and even then half is eliminated, causing blackening of your stools or constipation. Avoid drinking regular tea with meals as this blocks the uptake of iron and other minerals. Vitamin A deficiency has been found in women with heavy periods. By taking good levels of vitamin A, 92 percent of women found that their heavy bleeding was either cured or alleviated.[14]

Another study showed that supplementing with vitamin C (200mg three times a day) with bioflavonoids reduced heavy bleeding for 87 percent of the women tested.[15] Vitamin C with bioflavonoids helps to strengthen fragile capillaries, which can be a reason for heavy periods.

Take:
Multi-vitamin and mineral supplement designed for menopause
Beta-carotene (10,000iu)
Zinc citrate or amino acid chelate (15mg)
Vitamin E (300iu)
Vitamin C with bioflavonoids (1,000mg twice to three times a day)
Iron, as amino acid chelate or citrate (14mg)
Vitamin B complex (50mg of each B vitamin a day)

For maximum absorption, take the iron with the vitamin C at a different time from the other supplements.

Note:
Each nutrient represents the total intake for one day, so look at the contents of your multi-vitamin and mineral supplement and just add in any extras to the recommended amounts.

Herbs

Astringent herbs are usually used because of their ability to regulate blood loss. One such herb, shepherd's purse (*Capsella bursa-pastoris*) has been used successfully in clinical trials to prevent heavy bleeding. Other astringent herbs useful for heavy periods are ladies' mantle, yarrow, horsetail, golden seal, cranesbill, periwinkle and beth root. A good combination is equal quantities of shepherd's purse, cranesbill, yarrow and golden seal.

HOT FLASHES AND NIGHT SWEATS

These symptoms are experienced by more than eight out of 10 menopausal women, and are the reason why many turn to HRT. But if hot flashes are your main problem and you can get rid of them naturally, why take HRT?

Although hot flashes and night sweats have the same cause, and happen equally suddenly, they can have a different effect. While flashes can make you feel uncomfortably hot, on your face, neck or all over, sweats drench you, waking you up several times a night so you feel tired the next day. You may feel uncomfortable enough to change your nightclothes each time or even take a shower in the middle of the night. Despite this, women are often more self-conscious about hot flashes, believing that they are obvious to everyone else. But although there can be some redness or sweating, flashes are not always detectable and some women have told me that rather than getting hot flashes, they feel that their inner thermostat has changed so they just feel hotter all the time.

Practical changes can do a lot to ease the misery. When you get a hot flash see if there is a trigger that has caused it. They vary from woman to woman but common ones are spicy foods, caffeine and alcohol. Some women find that any hot drink can cause a hot flash. One woman who came to see me worked out that it was her nightly couple of glasses of red wine that were triggering night sweats, and she had to decide whether she preferred the red wine or the night sweats! For some women, stress or becoming anxious can start a sweat, which begins when adrenaline is released. This can cause night sweats too, if adrenaline is released following a drop in blood sugar in the middle of the night (see page 66). This is easily corrected by dietary changes.

To prevent stress from triggering hot flashes, scientists have asked women to practice deep, abdominal breathing (six to eight breaths a minute) twice a day, which has been found to halve the incidence of hot flashes. The breathing technique can also be used to make a hot flash more manageable when it starts.[16]

Another way to adapt is to wear several layers of clothes so that you can control your body temperature by taking off and putting on layers. At night, wear cotton nightclothes and use cotton sheets. This prevents moisture from being trapped by synthetic fabrics and turning into a cold sweat, which makes you wake up shivering.

Nutritional Therapy

Several studies show how vitamins can help control hot flashes and night sweats. Taking 800iu of vitamin E a day can significantly reduce hot flashes,[17] as can vitamin C with bioflavonoids.[18]

The primary function of vitamin C is to manufacture collagen, which helps to keep blood vessels healthy. Bioflavonoids, from citrus fruits, are closely associated with vitamin C. They are excellent at strengthening the small capillary blood vessels and this may be why vitamin C with bioflavonoids helps to control hot flashes and night sweats. Before menopause, estrogen keeps the blood vessels toned and prevents them from widening (a process called vasodilation) unless the body needs to cool down. The suggestion is that the vitamin C and bioflavonoids can compensate for the drop in estrogen levels that occurs at menopause by toning up the blood vessels, thus minimizing hot flashes.

So to eliminate hot flashes and night sweats, I would suggest that you take the following:

Multi-vitamin and mineral supplement containing boron (see page 103)
Vitamin E (800iu)
Vitamin C with bioflavonoids (1,000mg)
Probiotic (containing *Lactobacillus acidophilus* and other beneficial bacteria)

I have suggested that you also take a probiotic because isoflavones need to go through a process of fermentation before they can have a beneficial active estrogenic effect on your system. This can either happen because the food is already fermented (such as miso) or fermented by your own natural bacteria found in the digestive tract.

Note:
Each nutrient represents the total intake for one day, so look at the contents of your multi-vitamin and mineral supplement and just add in any extras to the recommended amounts.

Herbs

Many herbs are useful for hot flashes and night sweats, but two stand out: *Agnus castus* and black cohosh.

Agnus castus, also called Vitex or chastetree berry, is a member of the verbena family. It grows around the Mediterranean and Central Asia and was mentioned by Hippocrates for its benefits on the female reproductive system. It was originally used to decrease sex drive in men (especially monks), hence the name, but it may have the opposite effect on women's libido.

This herb is classed as an adaptogen as it helps to restore balance and is used where there is a hormonal deficit as well as in cases where there is an excess. It is also helpful for water retention and may have a beneficial effect on the thyroid.

This is one of the best herbs to take as menopause approaches, when you may still be having periods and ovulating (although not necessarily every month) and generally feel that your hormones are "all over the place."

Black cohosh (*Cimicifuga racemosa*), originally used by Native Americans, is also very effective in restoring female hormonal balance and relieving hot flashes.[19] A few years back, the British *Journal of Women's Health* stated that black cohosh "is a safe, effective alternative… for patients in whom estrogen replacement therapy is either refused or contraindicated."

Other herbs such as dong quai, licorice, sage and yarrow can also help counteract hot flashes and night sweats, so the best approach is to have a good mix of "menopause" herbs, with *Agnus castus* and black cohosh as staples.

Aromatherapy

Dilute 15 drops of Roman chamomile in 1 fluid ounce of carrier oil composed of two parts sweet almond oil and one part wheat germ oil.

Roman chamomile (not German chamomile) is an adaptogen, so it helps the body balance itself. Use the oil for a wonderful massage or simply sniff it during the day if you feel a hot flash starting.

LACK OF LIBIDO
Lack of Libido

Lack of interest in sex may have a lot to do with just feeling tired. Follow the recommendations for lack of energy to see if that makes a difference. When we are tired, the only thing we want to do when we get to bed is to go to sleep!

Lower estrogen levels, of course, are often blamed for lack of interest in sex. But is this true? It's interesting to note that while most women are told about

Phytoestrogens

Should you take phytoestrogen (isoflavone) supplements?

We know that women who eat a diet rich in phytoestrogens (soy, lentils etc.) have significantly fewer hot flashes[20] and other menopausal symptoms, but does this mean that taking phytoestrogen supplements also helps with hot flashes?

A whole food, containing fiber and other substances, behaves very differently in the body than a concentrated supplement. Isoflavones are extracted from soy or red clover by washing with alcohol and the isoflavones that are alcohol-soluble can be extracted. The alcohol is evaporated and the remaining isoflavone residue is sold as a supplement. Normally 40mg of isoflavones are recommended per day.

This whole idea of taking phytoestrogen supplements for menopause has exploded over the last several years and become a confusing minefield of information. What do you believe, do they work and are they safe? So let's ask a few questions.

Do phytoestrogens supplements help with hot flashes?

The weight of evidence seems to suggest that taking soy or isoflavone supplements helps with hot flashes by reducing them by about 45 to 50 percent,[21] although some studies have shown no benefit at all.[22] This is one of those situations in which I would suggest you try them and see if they work for you.

Where does red clover fit into this?

Red clover is a member of the legume family and has been used in agriculture for many years to improve the soil before another crop is planted. The flowers of the red clover have also been used for centuries by herbalists and are traditionally used as a treatment for skin problems, bronchitis, whooping cough and as an anti-spasmodic.

Red clover contains all four types of isoflavones (see page 54). At the moment some research shows no difference between women taking isoflavones derived from red clover for hot flashes and night sweats and women taking a placebo,[23] while one recent study published in *Maturitas* has shown a significant benefit.

continued

Are phytoestrogen supplements safe?

This is where I think you need to be cautious. Traditional cultures have eaten phytoestrogens in the form of soy, lentils, chickpeas, grains and other foods for thousands of years, but the use of phytoestrogens in tablets or capsules is relatively new. Nobody knows yet what the long-term effects of taking supplements like these might be. Supplements never offer the same beneficial effects that foods can. Foods contain a variety of different elements, including fiber, water and nutrients that do not appear in dried supplements. We found out, for example, that removing the active ingredients from herbal products and making them into pharmaceutical drugs brought with them a whole host of side-effects that simply did not occur when the herbs were taken whole. The problem is that we do not know if the same holds true here.

Red clover is not normally consumed in the same way as other phytoestrogens such as soy, where it is part of a traditional diet. The hormonal effects of red clover first came to light in the 1940s when it was noted that problems had arisen in female sheep that were grazing on red clover in Western Australia. The sheep had developed cystic ovaries, endometriosis and infertility. Analysis of the clover showed several phytoestrogen compounds.[24]

This has not been shown to be a problem in humans but until further research is conducted on the long-term effects of taking isoflavones from either red clover or soy, I would suggest that you just take them for a short while (up to six months) to help with the menopausal symptoms. At the same time, however, you should also make changes in your diet and start to include phytoestrogens in your cooking.

One phytoestrogen supplement is sold with the suggestion that it can increase breast size. It may have no effect, but if it does it must be stimulating the breast tissue. So for women with a history of breast cancer, I would suggest that you avoid concentrated phytoestrogen supplements until the research is conclusive (see chapter 9) and use traditional herbs to eliminate the hot flashes. It is very difficult to consume too many phytoestrogens in the diet and it is thought the foods actually have a protective effect on the breasts because of other substances that are also in the food (see page 161), but it is easy to take too many isoflavones when you can swallow them in capsule form.

falling levels of estrogen and progesterone, not much mention is made of testosterone. This is the "male" hormone linked with male characteristics such as deep voice and body hair, but it is also connected to drive and motivation. But women have testosterone circulating in their bodies too. It is produced by the ovaries and some women who have had their ovaries removed will often complain of lack of sex drive.

And it has been found that as we enter menopause, the level of this hormone can drop. But some women actually register an increase in testosterone at this time and feel their sex drive has actually increased, not fallen at all.

For other women, a lowering of libido may be caused by changes with age rather than menopause and can affect both men and women. Also it is important that your adrenal glands are not being overworked through stress or blood sugar fluctuations because they produce androgens, which are the male hormones.

Nutritional therapy

Make sure that you are not following a low-fat or no-fat diet as our sex hormones are manufactured from cholesterol. Include essential fatty acids in your diet in the form of nuts, seeds and oily fish.

Take:
Multi-vitamin and mineral supplement designed for menopause
Magnesium (300mg a day)
Zinc (15-30mg a day)
Vitamin B6 taken as 50mg pyridoxal-5-phosphate (one a day)
Flax seed oil (1000mg a day)

Note:
Each nutrient represents the total intake for one day, so look at the contents of your multi-vitamin and mineral supplement and just add in any extras to the recommended amounts.

Herbs

Herbs can be helpful for increasing sex drive. American ginseng is a good herb for increasing energy levels and can help with sex drive. It has been noticed that St. John's wort (*Hypericum perforatum*), which is used to help with depression, can also be helpful to increase libido.

If you are already taking medication, such as an antidepressant, you need to speak to your doctor before starting St. John's wort. It has been suggested that it can stop the contraceptive pill from working properly and there are concerns about interactions with other drugs, such as those for heart problems, blood clots, epilepsy, migraines and also drugs prescribed after organ transplants and for HIV treatment.

Ginkgo biloba can also be a good herb to try because of its enhancing effect on circulation. Having a good supply of blood to the sex organs can help to increase sexual stimulation and sensation. Damiana (*Turner aphrodisiacal*), a herb that is grown in Central America and Mexico, has been traditionally used by women and is best taken as a tincture before sex or once a day for a while to increase your sex drive.

Aromatherapy
Add 7 drops of damiana and 7 drops of geranium to a carrier oil. Damiana is a well-known herbal aphrodisiac.

MEMORY/CONCENTRATION
Poor memory, lack of concentration, impaired hearing and ringing in the ears are often caused by an obstructed blood supply to the brain. But this may be a problem to do with age rather than hormones. Brain cells alone account for 25 percent of the body's total oxygen consumption, so if there is any restriction in circulation then blood supply to the brain may not be as effective as it once was. As we age, we can also experience dizzy spells, as well as cold hands and feet, often a result of poor blood circulation.

With memory, as with sexual and bone health, it's another case of "use it or lose it." It is important that you keep mentally active. It is similar to our muscles. If we were bedridden for a number of months without using our muscles, we would find very difficult to walk when we finally got up, as our muscles would have began wasting away. The more we use our brains, the more interconnections we make and the easier it is to remember and concentrate.

Nutritional therapy
The hardening and narrowing of the arteries can be the cause of this reduced blood supply to the brain, so it is important that we keep the saturated fat content of our diet low. This hardening (arteriosclerosis) is caused by an accumulation of fats and the build-up of cholesterol in the arteries, which causes them to narrow and so restrict blood flow. The process is similar to the

furring up of a pipe, with the opening becoming smaller and smaller as the deposits increase.

Make sure you are eating well. Include fresh fruit and vegetables in your diet to keep your arteries healthy, as well as plenty of phytoestrogens, for they are not only helpful for hot flashes, but it has also been shown that eating a phytoestrogen-rich diet over a 10-week period compared to a low soy diet brought about significant improvements in both short-term and long-term memory.[25] Don't forget generous amounts of oily fish, which contain Omega 3 fatty acids. These contain essential components of brain cell membranes and can help age-related memory changes.

We know that the mineral boron is important for good bones because it helps the metabolism of calcium, but it is also important for good function and mental performance.[26]

Take:
Multi-vitamin and mineral supplement containing boron
Vitamin C (1,000mg a day)
Vitamin B6 (50mg a day)
Vitamin E (300iu a day)
Magnesium (300mg a day)
Selenium (100mcg a day)

Note:
Each nutrient represents the total intake for one day, so look at the contents of your multi-vitamin and mineral supplement and just add in any extras to the recommended amounts.

Herbs
The herb ginkgo biloba is now believed to have a rejuvenating effect on the brain. Several clinical trials have shown that it helps to enhance learning ability, concentration and memory. It also helps to improve blood flow to the head, increase the supply of glucose and oxygen that the brain needs to create energy, prevent blood clots and protect the brain cells against damage.

Research is also continuing with ginkgo to see whether it can delay mental deterioration or help alleviate Alzheimer's disease or dementia.

PAINFUL PERIODS (DYSMENORRHOEA)
Your periods can change as you get nearer to menopause. For some women they get heavier, and for others they get more painful.

First make sure there is no other underlying cause for the pain (such as endometriosis or infections). Endometriosis is where the lining of the uterus(the endometrium) grows in places other than the uterus itself. These tissues bleed during periods and cause severe pain. When you have checked that there is no organic cause, natural remedies can make a real difference to painful periods.

Nutritional therapy

Both magnesium and calcium work as muscle relaxants so it is worth supplementing with them. Get a good multi-vitamin and mineral supplement with a reasonable amount of calcium, then add the extra amounts below and see if that is sufficient. If you are still having pain after a few weeks you may need to add in extra magnesium with a supplement. Reduce your intake of animal foods, especially dairy products, to keep the arachidonic acid production under control. Arachidonic acid is a substance that encourages the production of hormone-like substances called prostaglandins. The prostaglandin that is produced from saturated fats is PGE2, a highly inflammatory substance that can cause swelling and pain and, in some cases, can thicken the blood itself. It can also trigger muscle contraction and constriction in the blood vessels, which can increase period pains, endometriosis-related cramps and the spread of endometrial tissue. Adding in essential fatty acids such as flax seed and oily fish can help with the pain.

Take:
Multi-vitamin and mineral supplement designed for menopause
Magnesium (300mg a day)
Flax seed oil capsules (1,000mg a day)
Vitamin E (300iu a day)
Vitamin C with bioflavonoids (1,000mg, two a day)
Zinc citrate (15mg a day)

Note:
Each nutrient represents the total intake for one day, so look at the contents of your multi-vitamin and mineral supplement and just add in any extras to the recommended amounts.

Herbs

Some herbs can help to relax muscles and stop abdominal cramps, while others help to promote the balance of female hormones. The wonderfully named cramp bark, for example, is an excellent antispasmodic and muscle relaxant. It is useful to combine a muscle relaxant like this with a good hormone balancer like *Agnus castus*, which addresses the cause of the pain.

Skin problems

Skin problems such as dry skin, eczema, psoriasis, acne, itching and skin rashes can often be attributed to a poorly functioning liver. Your liver is the waste-disposal unit of the body, not only for toxins, waste products, drugs and alcohol, but also for hormones. Food allergies have also been linked with skin problems so it would be worth looking to see whether anything you eat or drink may be causing the problem.

Nutritional therapy

The skin is an important part of this detoxification process. Sweating is essential for eliminating waste products, such as salt (sodium chloride), urea and nitrogenous waste through your skin. It also controls your body temperature because the evaporation of sweat from the surface of your skin has a cooling effect.

If you have skin problems, it is important to make sure that you eat as healthily as possible, avoiding fatty foods and those with additives, artificial sweeteners, colorings and chemicals in general. Make sure that you drink enough liquid (at least a quart a day) in the form of water or herbal teas. Include plenty of foods that contain essential fatty acids such as oily fish, nuts, seeds and oils, as a deficiency of these essential fats can have a direct effect on the skin.

Zinc is one of the most important nutrients for the skin, so it needs to be taken as a supplement.

Take:
Multi-vitamin and mineral supplement designed for menopause
Zinc (up to 30mg a day)
Vitamin B complex (containing 100mg of each B vitamin a day)
Flax seed oil (up to 1,000mg a day)

Note:
Each nutrient represents the total intake for one day, so look at the contents of your multi-vitamin and mineral supplement and just add in any extras to the recommended amounts.

Herbs

It is important to support your liver, so use the herbs that can help to cleanse it, milk thistle and dandelion. Herbs that work specifically on the skin include burdock root, which is useful for dry and scaly skin and eczema; it also been used to control dandruff. Licorice and German chamomile can be applied directly to the skin to help to calm it while you make the dietary changes that will have a long-term effect.

SLEEP PROBLEMS

Sleep problems can be quite different from insomnia. I see many women who have no difficulty in getting off to sleep but find themselves waking again. This can happen just once in the early hours of the morning or a number of times throughout the night. In either case, it may be a struggle to get back to sleep again.

This can be a common symptom at menopause, because of night sweats. If you are waking during the night because you are sweating, then your sleep will be disturbed and you will feel tired the next morning. It is important to use the recommendations for controlling hot flashes/night sweats first. If that does not work, you may have a more general sleep problem.

Insomnia should be tackled physically and mentally. Sometimes we are not sleeping because our minds are so active, and our thoughts are just going round and round. It is important to look at the dietary side too, as that is the easiest to control. Your sleep problems may be solved by adjusting what you eat and drink. If not, then it is time to take control of your mind.

Before going to bed have a relaxing bath with essential oils such as bergamot, lavender and chamomile. There are a number of good bath oils available in the shops that are already made up. Learn a relaxation technique that you can use in bed such as tensing and relaxing each part of your body in turn. Or try a visualization technique. Imagine yourself on a beautiful beach with the warm sun on your skin, soft sand under your feet, blue sky, clear water and with fragrant scent all around you from wonderful colored flowers. In the distance you can hear the sounds of birds and there is a gentle breeze in the palm trees. You have nothing to do and no cares in the world – just let yourself go. You can tape the visualization to play while you go to sleep, or you can buy a prerecorded relaxation tape.

Because our mental and physical states are so intertwined, they feed off each other, positively and negatively. If something is worrying us, our bodies become tense and unable to relax. This makes sleep more difficult, which in turn makes us even more stressed. If something physical is stopping us from sleeping, we feel worried and agitated, and then our bodies become even more tense and tight.

Nutritional Therapy

First, have a look at what you are eating and drinking during the day. Cut out all the stimulants such as tea, coffee, sugar, chocolate etc., and make sure you eat little and often; avoid going over three hours without food. Some women find themselves waking up at three or four o'clock in the morning, sometimes quite abruptly and with palpitations. This is caused by the blood sugar level dropping during the night. As the blood sugar level gets low, the body will release adrenaline into the blood stream to try and correct this imbalance. So at three or four in the morning there is a huge surge of adrenaline and you wake up, not knowing what's caused it.

Have a cup of chamomile tea before going to bed to help with the sleep problems.

Magnesium is known as "nature's tranquilizer," so it is a good mineral supplement for helping with sleep problems. You could take one dose about an hour before going to bed. If you take B vitamins try to take them in the early part of the day, not after lunch. A number of women I have seen who have taken B vitamins to increase their energy levels found they couldn't go to sleep when they took them in the afternoon or evening. If you suffer from restless legs in bed then I have found both magnesium and vitamin E to be very helpful.

Take:
Multi-vitamin and mineral supplement designed for menopause
Magnesium (250mg a day)
Vitamin E (300iu a day)

Note:
Each nutrient represents the total intake for one day, so look at the contents of your multi-vitamin and mineral supplement and just add in any extras to the recommended amounts.

Herbs

Herbs really come into their own here because they are so effective at helping us to relax naturally. Valerian has been used for centuries to help with sleep problems and its powers to help insomnia and improve sleep quality have been confirmed in studies. Ordinary sleeping pills can leave you feeling hung over and sleepy in the morning but valerian doesn't usually have this inconvenient side-effect at all. It is classed as a sedative in herbal medicine and can be used to reduce tension and anxiety and promote natural sleep.

Passion flower (passiflora) is another good herb for helping you sleep. It is thought that this herb contains alkaloids that work directly on the central nervous system to ensure restful sleep. It can be combined with valerian to give a very effective remedy for sleep problems without an addictive effect.

Blackboard technique

This is a good way of getting off to sleep. It's a variation on counting sheep – but much more effective.

• Lying in bed with your eyes closed, imagine a blackboard. Picture yourself with a piece of chalk in one hand and an eraser in the other.
• Draw a large circle. Inside the circle put the number 100.
• Use the eraser to rub out the number but be careful not to rub out the circle. When you have done this, write the number 99, rub it out as before and continue indefinitely.
• Even if you realize that you've gone back to thinking again, just stop and start from the last number you can remember.

The mind loses interest with this routine and eventually shuts down. As you do this exercise each night you should find yourself going to sleep more and more quickly because the mind becomes bored with the routine sooner. It can get to the point that you only have to think about the blackboard and the mind tells you, "Oh no, not again, sleep is preferable to this." If you wake in the night, do the blackboard technique or go to the bathroom and then come back to bed and do it.

STRESS INCONTINENCE

Stress incontinence is the leaking of a small amount of urine when you laugh, cough, sneeze or run. It can be embarrassing and inconvenient and women often don't even want to tell their doctors about it. It is thought to be linked to menopause because estrogen helps to keep the sphincter muscle at the base of the bladder tight. As estrogen declines, the muscle can become weak.

Kegel exercises (see page 195) can strengthen the pelvic muscles, including those of the vagina. These exercises can be done at any time because nobody knows you are doing them.

If you need extra help, vaginal cones containing small weights may help. They are inserted into the vagina in the same way as a tampon and by using them regularly you can gradually increase the strength of your pelvic floor and vaginal muscles. Some women find them easier than pelvic floor exercises, partly because they are fairly effortless, but more importantly because they automatically work the right muscles in the pelvic area. Pelvic floor exercises are only effective if they are done properly.

The cones work in exactly the same way as weight-training at the gym, only in this case the improvement is restricted to the pelvic area. The idea is to start with a small weight and keep it in place for about 15 minutes a day, while standing upright. As your muscle tone improves, you can progress to heavier weights. You should expect to see a difference in between eight and 12 weeks.[27] Once you have noticed an improvement, then you can maintain the muscle tone by using the cones two or three times a week.

Note:
If you have trouble obtaining the cones, contact me directly (see page 236). The vaginal cones should not be used during a period, or if you are suffering from a urinary tract infection or thrush.

Nutritional therapy
Eat well and follow the recommendations in the chapter on nutrition so that you are making the most of your own circulating estrogen to keep the muscles taut.

Vitamin C is important in stress incontinence because it produces collagen. Collagen gives skin its elasticity and can also help to retain the elasticity in the urinary tract and so prevent leakage or stress incontinence.

Take:
Multi-vitamin and mineral supplement designed for menopause
Vitamin C (1,000mg three times a day)

Herbs
Ladies' mantle (*Alchemilla vulgaris*) and horsetail (*Equisetum arvense*) are both useful herbs, as they are specifically indicated for stress incontinence.

VAGINAL DRYNESS
As the hormone levels change at menopause, the vagina can be affected. There is a tendency for the vaginal walls to become narrower and thinner and for the level of natural secretions accompanying sexual arousal to fall. This can make intercourse uncomfortable and is another one of those situations where you lose it if you don't use it. During lovemaking and orgasm, blood circulation is

increased in the vagina and this can revive the vaginal tissues. It is important to keep up a good intake of essential fatty acids in your food and not to go on a "no-fat" diet, as you need the lubrication from these oils

You might also need to apply a natural lubricant. One that I recommend is a New Zealand product called Sylk (available over the Internet). It is a natural, water-soluble lubricant derived from the kiwi fruit vine, which alleviates dryness by stimulating your own natural secretions. Sylk does not contain any hormones, drugs or animals products. It is also greaseless, non-sticky, stain-free and safe to use with condoms if you need a contraceptive.

If you reach the point where you cannot have intercourse at all because penetration is so painful, you need to take more drastic action. My suggestion would be to ask your doctor for a cream or suppositories containing estrogen. There are a number of different types made up of different kinds of estrogens. The least carcinogenic of these is estriol, so my recommendation would be to ask for a product containing this.

The cream or suppository is inserted directly into the vagina with an applicator to soften and tone the vagina, making intercourse more comfortable. The usual recommendation is to use it once a day for two weeks and then twice a week. When you get to this stage, use vitamin E vaginally (see below) a couple of times a week on the days when you are not using the estrogen product, together with lubricant when needed. If this is successful, cut down until you are using estrogen only once a week. Then see how you get on without the cream or suppositories to test whether the natural approach works on its own.

Changing your diet to include more phytoestrogens can also help. Foods such as soy or flax seed can change the cells of the vagina so that it becomes softer and more moist.[28]

Nutritional therapy

Vitamin C is important for vaginal dryness as it builds up collagen, which can give the vagina some elasticity. If the walls become less elastic they will not be able to stretch comfortably to accommodate an erect penis, so making intercourse painful.

Vitamin E is equally helpful. One study showed that just 400iu taken daily for between one and four months improved vaginal dryness in 50 percent of women.[29] It can also be used internally inside the vagina every night for about six weeks to help relieve dryness (but make sure you buy yeast-free capsules).

Herbs

Herbs such as *Agnus castus* which help to normalize the hormones at menopause will be useful. Motherwort can help by restoring thickness and elasticity to the vaginal walls. The Chinese herb dong quai is also useful for vaginal dryness.

WATER RETENTION

This is a common symptom for many women who suffer swelling and bloating and often it is worst just before a period. It can be so bad you may have trouble getting rings on your fingers and shoes on your feet.

Nutritional therapy

Your first instinct may be to limit the amount you drink. This is a mistake. In fact it's the opposite of what you actually need to do. You should drink more water, because if you limit your intake your body will think there is a shortage and try and retain what water you have, hence the swelling.

Reduce your intake of salt, including hidden salt in convenience foods. Table salt is sodium chloride and sodium is a mineral that affects your body's ability to balance water retention and blood pressure. Another mineral, potassium, works with sodium to regulate water balance and normalize heart rhythm. The more sodium you consume, the more potassium you need to counteract this effect. The World Health Organization recommends a maximum of 6 grams (1 rounded teaspoon) of salt a day. This supplies us with 2,400 milligrams of sodium. We only need 500 milligrams of sodium a day to keep us healthy.

Sodium is found naturally in all fruits, vegetables and grains and is already present in most ready-prepared foods, including salad dressings, cookies, bread, sauces and even canned vegetables. Most people end up eating about 9 grams of salt a day and it is easy to consume too much without realizing it. One burger in a bun can contain 6 grams, two slices of whole grain bread 1.2 grams and a slice of cheese and tomato pizza 5.3 grams. Two slices of bread contain more salt than an individual-size bag of potato chips.

We also consume sodium as sodium nitrate, which is the preservative used in meat, and as monosodium glutamate, the flavor enhancer, used extensively in convenience and Chinese food.

If you have a high salt intake, you could be carrying around an extra 4 pounds in excess weight due to water retention. A 1998 British government report on nutrition and heart disease by the Committee on Medical Aspects concluded that the reduction of salt in the diet by a third could save at least 34,000 lives a year. The usual first line treatment for high blood pressure is diuretics, which work by preventing the reabsorption of sodium and potassium. Doctors also recommend that we lose weight, take regular exercise, cut down on alcohol and stop smoking.

Many women who suffer from water retention will turn to diuretics. Diuretics will increase the rate at which you lose fluids but you will also lose vital minerals which will be flushed out of your body at the same time. Potassium is one of the minerals that you may lose but it is vital in the correct functioning of your heart.

Omega 3 oils should also be taken as they help your body to produce hormone-like regulating substances (prostaglandins) which enable your kidneys to eliminate water.

Take:
Multi-vitamin and mineral supplement designed for menopause
Vitamin C (1,000mg twice a day)
Flax seed (1,000mg twice a day)
Vitamin B6 (50mg a day)
Vitamin E (300iu a day)
Magnesium (150mg a day)

Note:
Each nutrient represents the total intake for one day, so look at the contents of your multi-vitamin and mineral supplement and just add in any extras to the recommended amounts.

Herbs

Dandelion (*Taraxacum officinale*) is a natural diuretic that allows fluid to be released without losing vital nutrients at the same time. Dandelion itself contains more vitamins and minerals than any other herb and is one of the best natural sources of potassium. Dandelion also helps to improve liver function so it can be useful for general detoxification and elimination of hormones.

The whole of the dandelion plant can be used therapeutically. The leaves have the greatest diuretic effect, while the root has a stronger action on the liver. This is one example of how using a whole plant rather than just parts of it can be important.

Parsley, rich in vitamin C, is also useful as a diuretic. If used to help reduce water retention, it should be taken in the tincture form for the most effective results.

It is also important to make sure that your hormones are in balance. Use normalizing herbs such as *Agnus castus* and black cohosh.

Aromatherapy

Fennel is very effective in countering water retention. Add 10 drops to a warm bath and soak in it for 15 to 20 minutes.

CHAPTER 9

Your Breasts at Menopause

Fear of breast cancer is very real for many women. Most of us know someone who has had breast cancer and endured what is often traumatic treatment. Many of us would admit it is our biggest dread. One in nine American women will develop breast cancer at some point in their lives; over 180,000 new cases are diagnosed each year, with over 40,000 women losing their lives.

As we get older, the statistical chances of developing breast cancer increase. Like most cancers, breast cancer is largely a disease of older women, with around 80 percent of cases occurring after menopause. The best way to protect ourselves is to be armed with information about the ways in which we can help ourselves, and that is what I aim to provide here.

Risk factors

No one knows for certain what causes breast cancer. However, research does indicate that some women seem to be more at risk than others. Many factors have been linked to an increased risk of breast cancer, and although some of them are outside your control, many are not. They include:

• obesity – linked to fat cells producing estrogen
• the Pill – but only if you start taking it at a very young age and stay on it for more than four years
• high intake of alcohol – increases estrogen because of the effect on the liver
• exposure to pesticides or radiation
• high saturated fat intake
• did not breastfeed
• family history – women who have close female relatives with breast cancer are more at risk than others. But this risk may not be as great as was previously thought. Four out of five women who have a mother and/or sister with breast cancer will not develop the disease. And eight out of nine women diagnosed with breast cancer do not have any close relatives with the disease.[1] A small minority of breast cancer cases, about 10 percent, seem to be linked to two faulty genes, BRCA-1 and BRCA-2.
• early periods and a late menopause – the two can go together and the combined effect is to increase the body's exposure to estrogen

• late babies – giving birth for the first time after the age of 35 is associated with a slightly higher than average risk of breast cancer
• getting older – women are at higher risk of breast cancer at and after menopause
• taking HRT – see page 31.

In some parts of the world, notably the Far East, breast cancer is not the major killer it is here in the West. Why? Japan has only one-sixth of the cases of breast cancer experienced here, yet when Japanese women move to the West and adopt a Western diet their breast cancer rate rises to Western levels.[2] Many experts think that the main factor is diet and this is borne out by the fact that as the traditional Japanese diet becomes more Westernized, cases of breast cancer are increasing. So changing your diet may be the best way to protect yourself from breast cancer.

There are a number of differences between the traditional Japanese diet and ours. The most striking is that the Japanese eat a good quantity of unsaturated fats, in oils and fish (which contain Omega 3 essential fatty acids known to inhibit tumor growth) while the Western diet is high in saturated fats from meat and dairy foods, which have never been important in Japan. The other main difference is their large consumption of soybean products, including tofu, miso (soybean paste), tamari (wheat-free soy sauce), tempeh and soy milk.

Cancer researchers believe that something in this diet protects the Japanese from certain cancers by controlling the overmultiplication of cells. Cells become cancerous when the normal process of growth and replication becomes haphazard and gets out of hand. With cancer, the cells do the job too well. The control mechanism that normally tells a cell to stop multiplying seems to be faulty and multiplication continues unchecked. Cells are programmed to die (a process called apoptosis) to make way for the new cells needed for development and maintenance. When your immune system is healthy and the cells are functioning well, growth and decay are kept in balance and cancer does not develop. When cells don't die, uncontrolled cell division can occur.

Surgery to remove tumors is based on the assumption that they are separate and independent manifestations of the disease, unconnected to the health of the rest of the body. The thinking is that if the lump – the diseased part – is removed in time, the cancer will be prevented from spreading. But although surgery cuts out as much of the growth as possible, it does not address the underlying cause, and the cancer may reappear at another site because the triggers are still there.

This theory is supported by research involving 5,500 breast cancer patients.[3] It demonstrates that mastectomy (radical surgery involving the removal of breast tissue and all lymph nodes in the armpit) guarantees women no greater chance of survival than if they have a lumpectomy (lump only removed) plus radiotherapy.

Conventional medicine, in many cases, focuses on treating the symptoms rather than the cause. There is a good analogy: imagine hard-working doctors busily mopping up water from an overflowing sink where both taps are on and the plug is in. They are frantically treating the never-ending "symptom," but the best approach would be to find and remove the cause!

The estrogen connection

Estrogen is your body's "builder," creating female characteristics such as breasts and helping to thicken the lining of the uterus ready to receive a fertilized egg, so it is easy to see how it could lead to an increased risk of cancer. It also explains why women who have had a surgical menopause (where the ovaries, which produce estrogen, are removed) seem to suffer less breast cancer and why women who start their periods early and have a late menopause (which extends their exposure to estrogen) are at higher risk. The use of estrogens in hormone replacement therapy is also linked to breast cancer and a number of studies show a 40 percent increase in breast cancer risk in women taking HRT.[4]

HRT increases the density of breast tissue, which naturally becomes less dense after menopause since it is no longer subjected to the stimulating effect of estrogen. It is thought that HRT affects natural cell death, causing a build-up of breast tissue and that this could be responsible for the increased risk of breast cancer.

It amazes me that the link between HRT and breast cancer has been known for almost 30 years but every few years we get the same newspaper headlines. In October 1997: "Don't panic plea over HRT link to cancer" (when news broke of a study showing that taking HRT increased the risk of breast cancer); in June 1999: "Cancer, the hidden peril for women taking HRT" (announcing that HRT increased the risk of breast cancer but it was less likely to be fatal, so don't panic). And then, in July 2000: "No need to panic over HRT risks," when the long-awaited Women's Health Initiative was abandoned five years into the eight-year study. But the "experts" in the U.K. argued that this latest study had involved the "wrong" group of women (who were between ages 50 and 79, older than most HRT users) and used the "wrong" HRT (a combination not available in the U.K.). Surely, over all those 30 years and the huge amount of data that has been collected, it can't all have been done on the wrong women and with the wrong HRT! To counter the criticisms, a study was published in *The Lancet* in September 2002 whose findings applied to all the forms of HRT used in Britain. This definitely showed an increased risk of breast cancer from taking HRT, and indicated that the risks did not outweigh any benefits.[5]

Obviously you can choose not to take HRT if you think it poses an unacceptable risk. What is more difficult is to escape being bombarded by estrogens in the environment and estrogen-like chemicals from pesticides and plastics called xenoestrogens (foreign estrogens). Some of the most dramatic effects of these chemicals have been seen in the wild. Fish have been found with both male and female organs, and in Florida, a group of male alligators developed very small penises and abnormal hormone levels. It transpired that there had been a massive spill of pesticide containing organochlorines in the lake where the alligators had hatched, releasing xenoestrogens that had feminized them. Hundreds of these organochlorines have been shown to cause cancer in humans and laboratory animals alike, and significant residues have been found in women with breast cancer, compared to those without.[6]

While studying breast cancer cells, Professor Ann Soto from Boston discovered just how potent this effect could be. One day the cancer cells started to divide and multiply as if estrogen were present. However, when the test tubes that contained the cells were changed, the cells stopped dividing. It turned out that the tubes contained nonylphenol, a synthetic estrogen similar to those used in paints, toiletries (especially skin creams), agricultural chemicals and detergents, which was seeping into the breast cell culture and stimulating the cells. Consider the implications if the moisturizer you have been using on your body – in particular your breasts – contained this chemical.

Two additional trends increase the effect of xenoestrogens on women. The first is that women are getting bigger. Xenoestrogens are lipophilic – which means that they love fat! They accumulate in fatty tissue, which is a particular problem for women, since they have a higher proportion of body fat than men. Added to this is the fact that simply being at the top of the food chain puts humans at greater risk. This is especially true for those who eat meat and dairy products, because animal products are likely to contain larger doses of xenoestrogens than food from other organisms. Meat from animals that eat smaller animals or contaminated grass, grain or water is likely to give more exposure than a plate of vegetables that has been sprayed with pesticides.

Secondly, increasing levels of xenoestrogens in the environment have coincided with earlier puberty. In 1900 the average age of onset was 15, but now girls as young as eight are growing breasts and pubic hair. As a result, foreign estrogens could have a major impact on women's health, not only by increasing their risk of breast cancer but also by contributing to other estrogen-linked conditions, such as fibroids and endometriosis.

What about mammograms?

A mammogram is a breast X-ray, and although it is commonly recommended for the detection of breast cancer, it has its negative side. First, X-rays can cause breast cancer, so ironically you could be exposing yourself to a test that can trigger the

---

Benign breast disease

Most breast problems are not cancerous. Many women complain of tender, swollen breasts and lumps that fluctuate with the menstrual cycle, a condition called fibrocystic breast disease. This can make the breasts so painful that their lives are seriously affected. Some women can't bear to hug their children and/or be hugged by their partners. Others can't wear tight clothing and some have difficulty sleeping because they can't find a comfortable position. In extreme cases, women may even opt for a mastectomy.

These benign changes in your breasts are telling you that your hormones are not functioning correctly. Improving your health by adjusting your diet and addressing any vitamin and mineral deficiencies you may have gives your body the chance to correct any imbalances. The recommendations are given in detail in chapter 8, but to summarize:

• Avoid drinks containing methylxanthines (coffee, black or green tea, chocolate, cola and even decaffeinated coffee) known to cause breast tenderness.

• Increase your intake of essential fatty acids by eating plenty of oily fish, nuts and seeds. Add supplements containing evening primrose oil, flax seed oil or fish oils.

• Try vitamin E supplements, which can also help to relieve the symptoms.[7]

Be breast aware

Although recent research has suggested that self-examination is ineffectual, more than 90 percent of breast tumors are first detected by women themselves, including cancers that can be felt but are not picked up by a mammogram. The main aim is to get to know your breasts. You need to become familiar with the shape and appearance of your breasts and get to know how they feel. Then you will notice if anything starts to change. If you are still having periods, the best time to check your breasts is when one has just ended. Spend time looking at yourself in the mirror, perhaps when undressing for bed or before getting into the bath or shower.

Standing in front of a mirror, raise each arm in turn above your head and move from side to side to get a good look at your breasts. Touch them to find out how they feel, and look at the shape and outline. Become aware of the position and shape of the nipple.

Lie on your back with your head on a pillow. Examine one breast at a time. Raise your right arm and put it behind your head. Using the tips of your left fingers, feel around the right breast in small, circular movements. Repeat on the other side.

Look for:
• any small lump in the breast or armpit
• a dimple or dent in the skin when lifting your arm
• any reddish, ulcerated or scaly areas of skin on the breast or nipple
• any bleeding or discharge from the nipple or moist, reddish areas that don't heal easily
• any change in nipple position – it might be pulled inward for example, or point in a different direction.

If you are concerned about anything you find, you should make an appointment to see your doctor at the same point in your cycle the following month. If your doctor examines you just before your period, it is more difficult to distinguish between what is harmless and related to hormonal fluctuations and changes that should be taken more seriously. If you are not having periods and you are concerned about anything, then see your doctor right away.

disease it is supposed to be detecting. Second, mammograms can result in false readings and unnecessary treatments. These false positives mean women may be recalled to have another mammogram and another dose of X-rays, and will have to undergo the emotional stress and anxiety the diagnosis causes.

There have been warnings since the early 1980s that screening seemingly healthy women might produce more cancer than it detects. This was borne out quite dramatically in a study in 1993. The Canadian National Breast Screening Trial examined more than 89,000 women over an eight-year period. Half of the women in the group received mammograms every year and the other half did not. The scientists found that among those women who had had mammograms there was a 52 percent increase in deaths from breast cancer compared to women who had not been screened in this way.[8]

This was followed in 1999 by the results of a massive 10-year study of 600,000 Swedish women, showing that mammograms do not reduce death from breast cancer. The researchers also warned of the possibility of mistaken diagnosis and that women might be subjected to unnecessary tests and surgery. They found that 100,000 women had been told they had cancer when they didn't, an alarming rate of one in six. Of these women, 16,000 had undergone a biopsy (where a needle is inserted into the breast to extract tissue for analysis) and more than 400 women had had unnecessary surgery, including mastectomy.[9]

Doubts were immediately cast on this study, possibly because some experts did not like what it said. So the data was independently re-analyzed, together with research from previous trials. The conclusion, which was published in *The Lancet* in 2001, was not only that "screening for breast cancer with mammography is unjustified,"[10] but that for every breast cancer death avoided, the total number of deaths increased by six. In other words, mammograms cause more deaths than they prevent.

When these findings were published, there was an immediate and widespread uproar. So the researchers went back and analyzed the data all over again, which simply reinforced the findings. "The results confirmed and strengthened our original conclusion," they wrote in *The Lancet* in 2001.[11] Dr. Richard Horton, the editor of *The Lancet*, concurred: "At present, there is no reliable evidence from large randomized trials to support screening mammography programs."

That should have been that, but because their conclusions were contrary to accepted wisdom, the authors of the study were asked to add statements to the article to lend support to breast screening before it would be accepted for publication. They refused, and the original results were published in full in 2001, in issue 358 of *The Lancet*.[12] However, an amended version appears in an update from the Cochrane Library, which collates the results of medical research (October, 2001), and this offers a different interpretation.

These researchers, who worked at the respected Nordic Cochrane Centre, had conducted a systematic review of all the randomized trials of mammogram screenings and came up with the conclusion that they weren't saving lives. Cochrane reviews are special reviews of scientific trials that are conducted to very high standards and certain protocols have to be followed. They carry much more weight than reviews that are conducted according to non-Cochrane protocols. If data had been subjected to a Cochrane review, you could have more confidence in the findings.

But once the conclusions came out, certain events were set in motion. Dr. Horton wrote a commentary in the October 2001 edition of *The Lancet* spelling out what had happened. He said that first of all the Cochrane Breast Cancer Group disowned the researchers' work and "found that their conclusions were unwelcome." The Cochrane Breast Cancer Group editors insisted that changes must be made to the review if it were to be published in the Cochrane Library. The researchers disagreed. So the editors added a statement to the results that lent support for screening and omitted data about the effects on subsequent treatment.

Dr. Horton points out that the main principles of the Cochrane Collaboration are to minimize bias in order to ensure quality, and that by interfering with the conclusions of the review, the academic freedom of the researchers is eroded and the credibility of science is open to question. The commentary mentions that the researchers had been concerned about "misleading statements" that had been added to the abstract and that important data had been omitted. The researchers had asked the Breast Cancer Group editors "to remove these two sentences," but the request was refused.

What *The Lancet* has done in a spirit of openness and transparency is to publish in full on its website (www.thelancet.com) the review by the researchers so that everybody can see the methods and analysis which led to those conclusions.

Women have to know that the judgments reached about screenings and treatments to which they will be subjected are based on sound scientific fact and not altered because somebody doesn't like the conclusion that was reached.

In addition, there are also practical problems involved in giving mammograms to pre-menopausal women and those on HRT. In the normal way, breast tissue becomes less dense after menopause, so it is fairly easy to spot subtle changes using a mammogram. This does not apply when the hormones are more active because the breast tissue is much more dense, which makes it difficult to get a clear picture. It has been suggested that women should stop taking HRT three weeks before they go for a mammogram.[13] By taking a break before screening, it may be possible to reverse the increased breast density caused by the HRT so that the mammogram is easier to read. Obviously it is better to avoid X-raying your breasts completely, if possible, or at least to keep mammograms to a minimum.

Ultrasound

It is also possible to scan the breasts using ultrasound. This has proved particularly useful for women who have dense breast tissue, which includes those who have not yet reached menopause and those on HRT. It is also used to investigate any problems detected by a mammogram. So why not skip the mammogram altogether? The main reason that ultrasound is not offered routinely is that it costs a great deal more than a mammogram. This is because it is much more labor-intensive, and each breast has to be scanned separately. If you are concerned about your breasts or feel a lump, you could opt for an ultrasound right away.

Preventing breast cancer

As with all things, prevention is better than cure. If you can keep yourself in good health, your body has a better chance of keeping the multiplication of cells under control. Cells have to multiply to grow and rejuvenate. You would die if that did not happen. But as we have seen, balance is important. Cells multiply for healthy reasons but when they overmultiply, the result can be cancer.

Taking an active role in trying to prevent breast cancer is important in a society where we are bombarded with environmental pollutants from different sources. You can help yourself by maintaining a strong and healthy immune system so that the growth and repair of cells is controlled. Diet is absolutely crucial because many cancers are thought to be linked to it. That is why it is important to eat foods that strengthen the immune system, to avoid foods that weaken it and to take steps to reduce your exposure to toxins at home.

Eat the right sort of fat

Scientists have found that the higher a country's intake of dietary fat, the greater the incidence of breast cancer.[16] Furthermore, "damaged" fats (those altered by deep-frying or processing for margarine, for example) increase the

The future of screening

Other screening include:

Hair tests

Professor Veronica James of the Australian National University has developed a test that aims to diagnose breast cancer from a single strand of hair. She has found that hair taken from a woman with the inherited breast cancer gene BRCA-1 has a different molecular structure than that taken from women who are free from breast cancer and who don't carry the genes likely to cause the disease.[14]

Electrical scanner

This hand-held machine has been approved by the Food and Drug Administration in the hope that it may reduce the number of unnecessary biopsies performed each year. The scanner distinguishes between benign and cancerous lumps by measuring electrical changes on the skin's surface. It has been known for many years that cancerous cells cause electrical disturbances and malignant tumors can be 40 times more conductive than benign tissue.[15]

Bra breast scanner

Researchers at De Montfort University in the UK have developed a bra worn for testing, which is packed with tiny electrodes that send small electrical currents through breast tissue. This avoids the use of X-rays and only takes a few minutes. Because tumor tissue is denser than healthy breast tissue, it is harder for electricity to pass through. By using sensitive measuring equipment it is possible to pick up the difference in tissue types, and as the electrodes are linked to a computer program, the bra also provides a 3-D image of the breast.

risk even more.[17] We know that chemically reactive atoms called free radicals (see page 56) are produced from "damaged" fats. We also know they can alter DNA and so contribute to cancer and heart disease. It makes sense then, to steer clear of the damaged fats that could trigger the onset of cancer.

It is also important to limit consumption of dairy foods such as milk, cheese and butter. These not only contain a high percentage of saturated fats but also large amounts of a growth factor IGF-1 (insulin–like growth factor) known to cause cell division in breast cancer cells.[18]

The Omega 3 oils found in oily fish and flax seed have been shown to inhibit tumor growth and help protect against breast cancer.[19] Monounsaturated olive oil can also lower the risk of breast cancer,[20] so it also has a role to play.

EAT PLENTY OF FRUIT AND VEGETABLES

Cancer rates are lower in people who eat the most fruits and vegetables. Cruciferous vegetables such as cabbage, broccoli and Brussels sprouts help to guard against breast cancer. They contain the compound indole–3–carbinol, which speeds up the elimination of estrogen, making it less dangerous. (Some breast cancers are estrogen–sensitive, so it makes sense that if levels of this hormone are reduced, the risk of developing breast cancer will fall.) The allium family of vegetables, which includes garlic, onions, leeks and spring onions, also has certain cancer–inhibiting properties. Garlic's sulphur compounds increase the activity of macrophages and T-lymphocytes, two components of the immune system that destroy tumor cells.

Fruit and vegetables are also good sources of antioxidants, which protect against cell-damaging free radicals. Antioxidant vitamins and minerals occur naturally in a wide range of foods. Vitamins A, C and E plus selenium and zinc can be found in carrots, pumpkins, green leafy vegetables, sweet potatoes, nuts, oily fish, vegetable oil and seeds. You may also decide that it is worth taking an antioxidant supplement, as research has shown that antioxidants can help to protect against a number of cancers.[21] Studies show that women with the highest levels of antioxidants, especially beta carotene, are 53 percent less likely to be diagnosed with breast cancer,[22] and antioxidants have even been linked with partial remission from breast cancer.[23]

INCREASE YOUR FIBER INTAKE

Fiber provides a very important protection against breast cancer as it determines how much estrogen you store and how much you excrete. If toxic waste products, including unwanted hormones, are not eliminated properly they may be stored in the body's fatty tissue, including the breasts – hence the link between chronic constipation and breast cancer.

Women who are worried about breast cancer are often told to watch their intake of saturated fat, which is good general health advice. What is not pointed out is that the fiber factor – increasing the amount of fruit and vegetables in the diet – can be much more important in preventing the disease. Soluble fiber (found in oats, and fibrous fruit and vegetables) is especially important as it binds estrogen, which is then excreted more efficiently.

EAT PHYTOESTROGENS

Phytoestrogens are a group of foods that contains substances that have a hormone-like action. In the human digestive tract, bacteria convert isoflavones (phyto-chemicals in soy, lentils etc.) found in these foods into compounds that have an estrogenic action, although they are not hormones. These phytoestrogens can help in many ways during menopause (see page 48). Most important of all, however, is the part they play in keeping the breasts healthy.

When cells are exposed to estrogen, normal orderly growth is disrupted. So why introduce yet more estrogen into your body? Because these plant substances can "fool" your estrogen receptors into accepting them, preventing other more powerful estrogens from locking on to the cells.

Unlike the estrogen your body produces, or that you take in HRT, phytoestrogens have a very weak estrogenic activity. The isoflavones they contain have only one thousandth of the potency of human estrogen, so they do not cause much breast cell stimulation.

These phytoestrogens fit into estrogen receptors in the breast but are too weak to stimulate the cells. What seems to happen is that these weak estrogens block the estrogen receptors in the breast and prevent cancer from developing. In simple terms, they stop the estrogens in the body from latching on.

Phytoestrogens also control the level of estrogen in the blood. They stimulate production of a protein produced by the liver called SHBG (sex hormone-binding globulin) which limits the action of sex hormones such as testosterone and estrogen, including estradiol, the most carcinogenic estrogen.[24] The fewer hormones there are circulating, the fewer there are available to stimulate breast tissue and possibly cause cancer.

Is it safe to take phytoestrogen (isoflavone) supplements?

Given the impressive record of phytoestrogens, you might assume that taking them as supplements can only do you good. But just because "some" is good, "more" isn't necessarily better. The idea of taking phytoestrogen supplements for menopausal problems is relatively new, and as yet there have been no studies on the effects of taking them for a long time. We know that it is safe to consume phytoestrogens such as soy, chickpeas and lentils as foods, and indeed research shows that eating these foods over long periods of time can protect against breast cancer.[25] The case may be very different for supplements.

Remember that women in other cultures eat phytoestrogens as part of their diet from an early age and for life. Swallowing isoflavones (concentrated phytoestrogens) from menopause onwards is not the same thing at all. At menopause we produce less estrogen naturally, so might adding in phytoestrogens in a concentrated form, even if they are weak estrogen, be a problem if a woman has an estrogen-dependent breast cancer or is at a higher risk of developing one?

There is also confusion about what happens if women on Tamoxifen (an anti-estrogen medication for breast cancer) take isoflavone supplements. Will the two compete against each other, and if so, what will happen? Nobody knows – research is inconclusive. Although one 1997 study on rats found that an isoflavone called genistein can protect against tumors,[26] others have shown the opposite effect. One study of premenopausal women undergoing surgery for a benign or cancerous breast tumor discovered that cell proliferation increased when they were given 45mg of isoflavones for 14 days.[27] A similar effect has been detected in laboratory trials, which found that red clover can stimulate breast cancer cells in the same way as estrogen.[28]

Another concern is the quality of phytoestrogen supplements. Not only are they made from different raw materials – soy germ, soy protein or red clover – but the amount of isoflavones they contain also varies enormously. One study, which analyzed 33 different brands, found that many had fewer isoflavones than claimed by the manufacturer. More worrisome, many of the supplements contained compounds the researchers could not identify, and so nothing is known about this cocktail.[29]

It is too big a leap to assume that phytoestrogen supplements will behave in the same way as phytoestrogens in food. The phytoestrogens in the foods are consumed alongside the vitamins, minerals, essential fatty acids, fiber etc. that are naturally contained in soy, for example. You are not just eating isoflavones on their own, which is what you are doing when you swallow an isoflavone supplement. And while it is very difficult to absorb too many phytoestrogens from food, it is very easy to overdose on supplements.

My advice to women with a history of breast cancer or an increased risk of the disease is to include phytoestrogens in their natural form as part of their diet, in soy milk, tofu, chickpeas, hummus, lentils and so on along with a variety of other good foods. Until further research is available I would not recommend taking phytoestrogens as supplements in any form, whether derived from soy or red clover.

What about using herbs if you have had breast cancer?

Women who have had breast cancer will often be advised not to take HRT, for obvious reasons, so is it safe to use herbs to control the hot flashes? Fortunately, there seems to be no reason why such women should not use black cohosh. Research shows that this does not stimulate the growth of MCF-7 cells, a breast cancer cell line.[30] In fact, when estrogen-dependent breast cancer cells were exposed to black cohosh, it actually slowed down the rate at which they multiplied, showing that the herb does not have estrogenic effects.[31]

Watch your weight

There are many reasons why being overweight is not healthy. Not only does it increase the risk of heart attack, high blood pressure and diabetes but it is also now known that being overweight and over 50 doubles your chances of developing breast cancer.[32]

Because fat cells are a manufacturing plant for estrogen, women who are overweight frequently have higher levels of the hormone, which puts them at greater risk of developing breast cancer. Overweight women also have lower levels of SHBG (sex hormone-binding globulin), a protein produced by the liver that binds sex hormones such as estrogen and testosterone and controls the amount circulating in the blood.

Where you pile on pounds matters almost as much as how many you put on. Researchers have found that women who put on weight around their middle (apple-shaped) are more likely to develop breast cancer than women with weight around their hips (pear-shaped). Doctors at the Harvard School of Public Medicine studying 47,000 nurses over a 10-year period found that those who had plump stomachs were 34 percent more likely to suffer from breast cancer than women with pear-shaped figures. When the researchers narrowed the study to focus on post-menopausal women who had never taken HRT, the apple-shaped women were 88 percent more likely to get breast cancer. Research has also shown that apple-shaped women are also more likely to suffer from heart disease, so it seems that carrying weight around the middle is not good for your health. If your waist-to-hip ratio is more than 0.8, you will need to take action! Here's now to calculate it:

1 Measure your waist at its narrowest.
2 Measure your hips at their widest.
3 Divide your hip measurement by your waist measurement to calculate the ratio.

For example:
34-inch waist divided by 37-inch hip = 0.9

This measurement is on the high side, possibly increasing the risk of breast cancer, so it would be worth aiming to lose weight by following the recommendations in Chapter 11.

Exercise

A fascinating study reported in the *Journal of the National Cancer Institute* showed that women who exercised for around four hours a week had a 58 percent lower risk of breast cancer than women who did not exercise, and those who routinely exercised for between one and three hours a week had a 30 percent lower risk.[33] The thinking is that regular exercise can modify hormonal activity in a beneficial way. It is known that extremes of exercise alter the menstrual cycle dramatically – many women athletes, for instance, do not have periods at all. So it is believed that moderate routine exercise suppresses the production (or overproduction) of hormones, reducing exposure. However, this needs to be a life change rather than a quick fling. Establishing exercise routines is important before, through and after menopause, to reduce the risk of breast cancer and osteoporosis (see page 106).

Can your clothing affect your breasts?

It has been suggested that wearing a bra can increase the risk of breast cancer by suppressing the lymphatic system, causing toxins to accumulate in the breasts.[34] The statistics from the bra study showed that women who wore a bra for more than 12 hours a day were more likely to develop breast cancer than those who wore their bras for a shorter time. Because this study was flawed in strict scientific terms, it is difficult to place too much emphasis on its results, but I think that sensibly we should give our breasts a chance to "breathe."

Avoid environmental toxins

This is really a case of "do the best you can," because you cannot control everything. Perhaps the best place to start is with food. Because breast cancer can be estrogen-driven, there are obvious concerns about the impact of xenoestrogens – harmful environmental estrogens from pesticides and plastics – on the body. More organochlorines from pesticides have been detected in women with breast cancer than in those who have benign breast disease.[36] The best advice is to eat as much organically grown food as possible and don't use pesticides in the garden.

Xenoestrogens come from plastics as well as pesticides, so try to buy fruit and vegetables loose or in cardboard containers rather than tightly wrapped in plastic (obviously you won't be able to avoid all contact with plastic). When you get food home from the store, remove any plastic packaging as soon as possible. Don't store food in plastic containers – use glass or china dishes with lids instead. Avoid using plastic food wrap too, especially in the microwave. Because xenoestrogens are lipophilic (fat-loving), they tend to migrate into

---

Microwave ovens

Just a word about microwaves because now almost three-quarters of households own a microwave oven. The microwave oven heats food by using high-frequency electromagnetic waves, similar to those in television. The molecules of the food agitate at over 2,000 times per second so that the food heats itself. The idea is that the metal oven is a sealed unit, microwaves cannot penetrate metal so they cannot escape. But there have been health concerns about microwave ovens because of the possibility that radiation could be leaking out during cooking. There are also worries that food cooked in a microwave may be inherently changed in ways we are not yet aware of.

Microwave cooking seems to destroy the cell walls of plant foods such as vegetables. Studies on microwaved carrots and broccoli show that the molecular structure is deformed, whereas in conventional cooking the cell structure stays intact.[35]

What this means is that the microwave process seems to encourage the production of harmful free radicals (see page 56) and that it is probably advisable to cook using conventional methods as often as you can.

---

foods with a high fat content, such as cheese, so it is important not to heat dishes containing dairy foods in plastic.

You can also strengthen your defense against xenoestrogens (bad) by including phytoestrogens (good) in your diet. Studies have shown that genistein, an isoflavone or type of phytoestrogen in soy, can inhibit the growth and development of breast cancer cells induced by pesticides.[37]

Look at the cleaning agents and detergents you use, too. Buy the brands that contain the fewest chemicals, so that you do not fill your home with unwanted toxins. Even though cleaning products may include only small amounts of chemicals, it is the cumulative and cocktail effect that may cause problems. Instead of air fresheners you could use an aromatherapy oil burner.

Other chemicals in everyday items used in the home have also been linked to breast cancer. Some of these chemicals are endocrine disrupters, which means that they can have a negative effect on our hormones. A report by the U.K. Consumers' Association in August 2002 detailed the dangers of seemingly harmless products that can remain in our bodies for years. This is an excellent report as it also names the manufacturers, so that you can tell whether the shampoo or shower gel you use, for example, contains these chemicals. The Consumers' Association listed a number of chemicals, including:

• artificial musks – used in perfumes and air fresheners
• bisphenol A – used in linings of food and drink containers, polycarbonate plastics used to make water bottles, food storage containers and babies' feeding bottles
• alkyphenols – used in some shampoos and shaving foams, paints and glues.

Toiletries and skin-care products

Awareness is even more important when it comes to toiletries, skin care and cosmetics, all products you put on your skin. Chemicals are absorbed through the skin (that is how HRT patches work) so anything you apply can enter your bloodstream. We cannot avoid all these harmful chemicals because of the nature of the society in which we live. But think about what you are putting on your body, and that means considering the face creams, suntan lotions, body lotions, hair-removing agents and anything else that you may use. Read the ingredients list. Ask yourself whether you could choose a more natural alternative to the brand you are using, particularly if you are using it around the breast area.

Your choice of deodorant, for example, could be crucial. Scientists are currently investigating the link between the use of deodorants and antiperspirants and breast cancer. Because these products are applied to the armpit, the theory is that the chemicals they contain may leach into the breast. Dr. Philippa Darbre from Reading University is investigating chemicals known as parabens, used as a preservative in many deodorants, to find out if they are implicated in the increasing number of cancers found in the upper breast near the armpit.

There are also concerns about aluminum in deodorants. This heavy toxic metal has been linked to dementia, and has been found in patches of cell damage in the brains of people with Alzheimer's. To avoid contamination, it is best to buy an aluminum-free deodorant from a health store.

I think it is better to avoid antiperspirants in favor of deodorants, which will not stop you from sweating, but will prevent any odor. After all, your body sweats for a reason. Sweating eliminates waste products such as salt (sodium chloride), nitrates and urea through the skin. It also controls your body temperature. The evaporation of sweat from the surface of your skin has a cooling effect on the body, useful when you are having a hot flash. If you use an antiperspirant, you prevent this natural process from occurring and are effectively hampering the elimination process.

★

Women often feel helpless in the face of what appears to be a rising tide of breast cancer. As we get older, more of our friends and relatives seem to become victims. I hope I have shown that there is a great deal that you can do in terms of prevention, both for yourself and your daughters. The major research studies reveal that diet is absolutely crucial and that what we eat is as important as what we avoid. It lies within the power of every woman to use this knowledge to prevent the disease. We can do something positive, and we should.

CHAPTER 10

Your Heart at Menopause

Apart from the prevention of osteoporosis, protection against heart disease is the main reason why many women have been encouraged to begin taking HRT. It was touted as *the* treatment that could decrease the risk, even though heart disease is not a "symptom" of menopause. It is true that as women get older their risk of cardiovascular disease changes. By the time women reach 50, they have half as much risk of heart disease as men. It is not until they get to the age of 75 that they have an equal risk. Unfortunately, we now know that far from protecting women's hearts, HRT may do quite the opposite.

As long ago as 1997, I stated that there was nothing to show that HRT would prevent heart disease. The evidence just wasn't there. So how did this belief come about? The first study to show that HRT seemed to have a protective effect on the heart and circulation was reported in 1985.[1] It followed the progress of a number of nurses, who were divided into two groups, depending on whether they took HRT or not. When those taking hormone therapy appeared to be less susceptible to heart attacks, doctors promptly began to prescribe HRT to menopausal women to protect their hearts.

The enthusiasm of the medical establishment for HRT was particularly unfortunate because the study was flawed. The best clinical trials are double-blind and placebo-controlled, which means that nobody knows who is taking the drug and who has been given a placebo, or dummy pill. In the 1985 trial, the scientists knew exactly who was on HRT and who was not.

This is important because it meant that a number of women who were at high risk of heart disease may have ended up in the non-HRT group, and that may have skewed the results. Conditions such as blood clots (thrombosis) and high blood pressure usually rule out HRT (see page 33), so it is unlikely that any nurse with a history of these problems would ever have been prescribed it.

The result was far-reaching. For more than a decade, HRT was prescribed in the belief that it would protect women's hearts. It was not until 1998 that results from the first randomized, double-blind, placebo-controlled trial – the HERS trial (Heart and Estrogen/progestin Replacement Study) – on the subject showed that there was no benefit in taking HRT for heart disease. The women in this study had already experienced heart problems and the HRT was given to see whether it would prevent a second attack. On the contrary, it found that women taking HRT were nearly three times more likely to have a clot in a vein.[2]

Although this caused some alarm, it was not enough to change prescribing practice because the women recruited for the study had already experienced heart problems and HRT was given in the hope that it could prevent a second attack. In fact, the reverse is true. In 2001 the American Heart Association (AHA) weighed up all the research available since 1998 and decided that estrogen should not be used to prevent heart disease, either for women who already had heart problems or for women who were trying to prevent them.[3] What they were effectively saying was that HRT does not prevent heart disease.

And then, in 2002, came the results of two long-awaited studies. The follow-up to the HERS 1998 trial was published, showing that women who already had heart problems had an increased risk in the first year of taking HRT.[4]

But the critics countered that these were women who already had a heart problem – what about healthy women taking HRT and the benefits to the heart? Well, the results of the first randomized trial to look at the effects on heart disease in healthy women taking HRT was published in July 2002. It is unbelievable to think that women had been told to take HRT to protect against heart attacks for all those years without anyone conducting a proper clinical trial to see whether it worked.

What the results showed was that apart from not protecting against heart attacks, HRT actually increases the risk of heart disease by 29 percent. The evidence was so conclusive that a long-term trial on combined hormone replacement therapy by the Women's Health Initiative was abandoned three years before it was due to end.[5]

Reducing the risk of heart disease

Heart disease is not just "one of those things." You are not struck down by a heart attack out of the blue, because your heart and circulation will have been unhealthy for some time. Heart disease is a degenerative disease, which means that problems have been building up for a number of years. And most experts agree overwhelmingly that these can be caused – or prevented – by your lifestyle.

What are the risk factors?

These are some of the factors that can increase your risk of heart problems. If you have any of them, you need to put into place all the
continued

recommendations, including dietary changes, supplements and exercise, given in this chapter.

- Family history of heart disease or stroke
- Smoking
- Too little exercise
- High cholesterol
- High blood pressure (even if controlled by medication)
- Diabetes
- High intake of saturated fats (in meat and dairy products)
- Stress
- Being overweight
- Earlobe crease. The link between an earlobe crease and heart disease has been known in Eastern medicine for hundreds of years, but it wasn't established by a clinical trial until 1983. Since then, 30 studies have confirmed this finding.[6] The earlobe usually receives a rich supply of blood, but if it is deprived of this, a crease develops. So an earlobe crease can be a sign of restricted blood flow through the heart.

The cardiovascular killers

A heart attack, which is also called myocardial infarction (or MI), occurs when an area of heart muscle is completely deprived of blood and the heart muscle cells die. A heart attack may result when plaque inside the heart arteries breaks open or ruptures, forming a clot that significantly blocks blood flow through the artery.

A stroke occurs when blood flow is blocked by a clot in a blood vessel (artery) that supplies blood to the brain.

Heartstopping

The connection between diet and heart disease is one of the best known in medicine. There are several factors that increase your risk of heart disease.

WHAT IS CHOLESTEROL?

Whenever you hear mention of the word cholesterol, it is always negative. But cholesterol is essential for life. It is manufactured in the liver and has a vital part to play in the structure of cells and the composition of certain hormones, particularly sex hormones. Your body makes all the cholesterol it needs in the liver and intestines, so taking in extra from foods that are naturally high in cholesterol is not necessary.

Your body is constantly striving for balance and if you eat a meal that raises cholesterol levels, it compensates by telling the liver to manufacture less. The mechanism is like a thermostat, switching the heat up if the temperature drops and turning it down if the house becomes too hot. To work efficiently, the system has to be well maintained and in good working order. And it can be misused, because you can override the thermostat. Your liver does not stop producing cholesterol altogether, so if you eat cholesterol-rich food continuously, it cannot compensate completely and the cholesterol in the blood remains too high.

Some of the cholesterol your body makes is absorbed directly into your bloodstream during digestion. It is carried to the cells by low-density lipoprotein (LDL or "bad" cholesterol) and then taken away to the liver to be excreted by high-density lipoprotein (HDL or "good" cholesterol). The balance of these two lipoproteins in the blood is far more important than the total amount of cholesterol. If the LDL ("bad") level is high, cholesterol will be deposited, and if the HDL ("good") level is low, it will not be carried away. The cholesterol may then accumulate on the artery walls (a process called arteriosclerosis). The arteries clog up, becoming narrow and hard, in the same way that deposits from hard water fur up pipes. The result? Heart disease.

When you have a medical check-up, it is definitely worth asking to have a lipid (fat) profile taken, especially if you have a family history of heart disease or stroke. Then if you know there is a problem, you can take action. This will give you four measurements: total cholesterol, HDL, LDL, and triglycerides (the form in which fat is stored in your body). Remember that a lipid test needs to be performed on an empty stomach, so schedule the test for first thing in the morning. Eat nothing before you go and drink only water.

Ideally, the total amount of cholesterol in the blood should be below 200mg/dl per liter. LDL should be below 130 and HDL above 35. Other experts have suggested that a better measurement is the ratio of your cholesterol to HDL. A ratio of 3:1 is considered to be good, 5:1 is normal and anything over that is high-risk.

HOMOCYSTEINE – THE "NEW" CHOLESTEROL

For years, cholesterol was considered the most significant dietary factor in heart disease, but now scientists are focusing increasingly on homocysteine.

Homocysteine can cause problems if it is not processed properly and remains high in the blood. Made from protein in the diet, it is a byproduct of an essential amino acid called methionine, which in normal circumstances is detoxified by the body. Because homocysteine is toxic, high levels contribute to the thickening and hardening of the artery walls, making the blood more likely to clot, damaging the blood vessels, and resulting in the buildup of fatty deposits, or plaque.

This effect was discovered in the 1960s, when researchers realized that children with a rare metabolic disorder that caused high levels of homocysteine usually died of blood clots and heart attacks. The autopsies showed that although these children had normal cholesterol levels, the damage to their arteries was virtually identical to that found in elderly people. The scientists then asked: "Could high levels of homocysteine be a risk factor for heart disease in adults?"

The answer from over 30 trials is a definite "yes," especially for those whose diet is low in B vitamins (especially B6, B12 and folic acid), which detoxify homocysteine, and high in protein, which creates it. So if you eat a high-protein diet, which is not good for your bones anyway (see page 95), and you are not getting enough of these three vitamins, you could be storing up trouble.

Luckily, it is possible to control homocysteine using a few simple and practical steps. If you have a family history of heart disease, ask for your homocysteine levels to be checked when you have a test for cholesterol. If these are high, you need to improve your intake of vitamins B6, B12 and folic acid, and have another test in three months" time. Research indicates that the best amounts to take to reduce homocysteine levels are 0.5-5mg of folic acid, 500mcg of vitamin B12, and 25-50mg of vitamin B6.[7] Simply adding these nutritional supplements to your diet makes it possible to lower your risk of heart disease.[8]

THE PROBLEM WITH IRON

A few years back, a pathologist named Jerome Sullivan from South Carolina set out to discover why men are more likely to die from heart disease than women. He had observed that women who'd had a hysterectomy had a higher risk of heart problems than women who hadn't. He also knew that postmenopausal women have a higher risk. He realized that hysterectomy and menopause have one feature in common – they stop women having periods. Why would this make a difference? Because when women menstruate, they lose iron – about 500mg a year.

Iron is a strange mineral. It is needed to make red blood cells and hemoglobin, to transport oxygen around the body. Without iron, new cells could not be produced and the organs would be starved of oxygen. So it is not surprising that until recently, scientists thought that the more iron you had, the better. But the negative side is that iron is continually stored as ferritin and rarely leaves the body. The only times you lose iron are during a period, childbirth, loss of blood through injury, or when you donate blood – and it is known that people who donate blood have a reduced risk of heart attack.[9] In contrast, men – who lose blood far less often than women – are at higher risk. Sullivan found that by the age of 45, a man has as much iron in his blood as the average woman of 70, and the same statistical risk of heart attack.

When Jerome Sullivan published his findings in *The Lancet* in 1981, the medical community was not impressed. They were still obsessed with producing drugs to lower cholesterol. Then, in 1990, the cardiologist John Murray, who had been studying African cattle herders, observed that none of the men over 50 had heart disease, even though their diet mainly consisted of whole milk – high in saturated fat and cholesterol. Whole milk is low in iron, so Murray proposed that maybe cholesterol becomes harmful when combined with iron's oxidizing effects. He decided to measure cholesterol's "stickiness" by giving extra iron for 60 days. The result was that more "bad" (LDL) cholesterol was produced in the body.

There is now a large body of evidence to suggest that LDL only damages the arteries when it becomes oxidized.[10] Stored iron plays a part in this by producing destructive free radicals. Free radicals speed up the aging process by destroying healthy cells and increasing the risk of heart disease. That is why it is crucial to get enough antioxidants in your diet and to reduce your iron intake.

There is no benefit from having excess iron, quite the opposite. Don't think that you should take it as a "tonic" when you are feeling tired or run down. Because it is not eliminated from the body, you will simply keep storing it. Only women who are anemic need extra, so get your hemoglobin and ferritin levels checked before you take more iron. If your ferritin level is high, choose food supplements without iron, buy non-fortified breakfast cereal and look carefully to see whether iron is hidden in foods such as bread or pasta before you buy them.

SATURATED FAT

Saturated fat can be detrimental to your heart because it increases the risk of atherosclerosis, where deposits of fatty materials are laid down in the arteries.

As well as limiting your intake of animal foods, including red meat, cheese and milk, it is important to avoid trans fatty acids, found in margarine and ready-made cakes and pastries. They are produced by hydrogenation so look for the words "hydrogenated fat" on the label before you buy that apparently healthy low-fat or polyunsaturated spread. Trans fats have been linked to an increased rate of heart attack and because they cannot be properly metabolized, they can end up being a bigger problem than saturated fats.

BEING OVERWEIGHT

Weight gain is another important factor in heart disease. The risk seems to increase if you are carrying more weight around your waist and stomach than round your hips and thighs, so in this respect at least, the pear shape is a good thing. However, it is important not to be complacent if you have always had this body shape. After menopause, fat distribution changes, and more can be deposited around the stomach. It is worth checking your measurements and taking action if your waist-to-hip ratio is more than 0.8 (see below), which means you may be at higher risk of heart disease, diabetes, osteoporosis and arthritis.

1. Measure you waist where it is narrowest
2. Measure your hips at their widest point
3. Divide your waist measurement by your hip measurement.

For example:
31-inch waist divided by 37-inch hip = 0.84

SMOKING

Although most smokers are aware of the threat of lung cancer, many fail to realize that they are also at high risk of heart attack and arterial disease, including "smoker's leg," which can endanger the limbs. Smoking thickens the blood, leads to blood clots and also raises blood pressure, increasing the risk of heart attack by 70 percent.

Heartwarming

There are plenty of positive things you can do to reduce the risk of heart disease. Eating sensibly and taking exercise are common-sense approaches worth taking at any time, but especially after menopause. Simple ways to improve heart health include taking more of all of these.

Eat more oily fish, nuts, seed and oils

The essential fatty acids in these foods are important for the prevention of heart disease. Inuits eat vast amounts of fat and yet they have an extremely low rate of heart disease because the fat comes from fish, which is known to be high in Omega 3 essential fatty acids. These Omega 3 oils have been found to lower cholesterol and triglycerides (fat stored in the body), decrease blood pressure, prevent blood clotting and raise HDL (the cholesterol remover), reducing the risk of hardened arteries. So include fish (especially oily fish) in your diet twice to three times a week and eat a handful of nuts or seeds every day.

Eat more phytoestrogens

In addition to their hormone-balancing function, phytoestrogens such as soy, chickpeas and lentils can help to lower cholesterol. Studies have shown that eating soy decreases levels of LDL ("bad") cholesterol and triglycerides (stored fats) and that the higher the initial cholesterol level, the greater the effect.[11] The Food and Drug Administration (FDA) now allows manufacturers to advertise the benefits of soy on food labels: the agreed wording is that 25 grams of soy protein a day may reduce the risk of heart disease as part of a diet low in saturated fat and cholesterol. Tofu contains approximately 12 grams of soy protein per 100 grams and two glasses of soy milk provide about 20 milligrams, so that is not an excessive amount to eat.

It is much better to consume soy protein that is contained naturally in foods such as tofu rather than soy protein concentrates or powders. Incidentally, up to 90 percent of the isoflavone content of the soy is removed in the extraction process in order to obtain the soy protein, so there would be minimal phytoestrogen benefit from using soy protein.

How soy has this effect on cholesterol is not yet known, although several theories have been put forward. The first is that soy encourages the excretion of bile acids (and therefore cholesterol) via the feces. Another is that because soy is a soluble fiber, it binds with some of the cholesterol and fat in the food you eat. The fiber passes out unabsorbed, so it keeps both of these under control. The third idea is that soy has an antioxidant effect. Genistein and daidzein, the isoflavones in soy, both have antioxidant properties and can help to reduce narrowing of the arteries.[12]

Although most research has focused on soy protein or isoflavone supplements, it is much better to eat phytoestrogens as part of your diet. Will these have the same beneficial effect on your heart? Yes, because a recent study of postmenopausal women found that eating phytoestrogens helps to increase HDL, the "good" cholesterol.[13]

Increase your antioxidant intake

Fruits and vegetables supply us with antioxidants, which can protect against heart disease by attacking the harmful free radicals that cause cell damage (see page 56). They are abundant in highly colored fruit and vegetables, and this may help to explain the French Paradox – the fact that despite their high consumption of saturated fat, heart disease is relatively uncommon in France. The secret seems to lie in their high consumption of wine.

Grapes contain an antioxidant called resveratrol, which decreases the stickiness of blood platelets and keeps blood vessels from narrowing. The highest concentrations are found in the skins of the grapes, which is why red wine (made from whole grapes) seems to be more effective than white (made from the flesh). Resveratrol has nothing to do with alcohol content and it seems that drinking red grape juice could be even more effective. Scientists have compared the effect of alcoholic and non-alcoholic red wines and found that the non-alcoholic version is actually better for the heart.[14]

In addition to eating sufficient fruit and vegetables, anyone with a family history of heart problems would do well to take a good antioxidant supplement. Vitamin E, a powerful antioxidant, has been studied extensively in relation to heart disease. It has been found that 100–400iu of vitamin E daily significantly reduces the risk of coronary heart disease and heart attacks. A study by scientists from Cambridge University and Papworth Hospital, published in *The Lancet*, found that taking a daily dose of vitamin E reduced the risk of heart attack by an astonishing 75 percent.[15] This is probably because it prevents the "bad" LDL from oxidizing (or going off) in the blood.[16]

Increase your fiber intake

There are two main types of fiber: soluble and insoluble. Insoluble fiber is found in whole grains and vegetables, while soluble fiber is found in fruits, oats and beans. Soluble fiber helps to control cholesterol because it binds with some of the cholesterol and fat in the food you eat.

Exercise

Brisk exercise that gets your heart beating faster than usual helps to keep it healthy. Besides keeping the cardiovascular system in good condition, exercise also seems to raise levels of HDL ("good" cholesterol) and lower LDL ("bad" cholesterol).

★

It is quite disgraceful that women have been told for many years that HRT can protect them from heart disease when the medical knowledge had been inexact and flimsy at best. The whole theory had been based on myths. Far from giving any protection, HRT in fact increases the risks of both heart disease and stroke. Fundamentally, there is no substitute for a "heart healthy" lifestyle. Of course this requires effort, because there is no quick fix when it comes to getting and staying healthy. But it does work, which is more than one can say for HRT.

CHAPTER 11

How to Control Your Weight and Your Moods

Menopause is good news for any woman who is struggling to lose those last few pounds. My message is to stop worrying, because some weight gain at this time is perfectly acceptable. As your ovaries reduce their production of hormones, your body fat acts as a manufacturing plant for estrogen, and the extra 9 to 11 pounds will serve you well.

Being too thin at this time of your life can be as unhealthy as being too fat. Ideally, women should have 25 percent body fat in contrast to men's 15 percent. Yet women face a lot of pressure from society, especially the media, to keep slim, and at its extreme, this can result in eating disorders such as anorexia and bulimia. Other women may spend much of their lives yo-yo dieting, which in the end completely distorts their attitude to food.

The extent of this obsession can be gauged by the fact that the U.S. diet industry has an annual turnover of $40 billion per year. The irony is that despite this emphasis on losing weight, statistics tell us that women are getting heavier, not lighter.

Why diets don't work

Dieting can be a losing battle. As you reduce your food intake or skip meals, your body puts itself on "famine alert." It gets the impression that food is scarce and therefore slows your metabolism to get the most from the small amount of food you are eating. So if you crash-diet for a week and then resume your usual food intake, you will be eating normally again but your metabolism will be slower, so you will end up putting on weight far more easily.

The famine effect also means that a punishing diet can actually increase your fat stores. If you lose weight quickly by restricting your intake and then start eating normally, a much higher percentage of food will be laid down as fat. Why? Because your body wants to build up those extra fat stores, in case a food shortage occurs again. So strange as it may sound, eating more of the right foods can help you to lose weight. And not only do you risk putting on more weight after coming off a diet but there is also a distinct possibility that you will need a more restrictive diet next time in order to lose weight. Then you are stuck in a vicious cycle of trying one diet after the other because the weight loss is not permanent.

The conventional approach to weight loss has been the idea of reducing calories. In scientific terms, a calorie is a unit of heat and the energy-producing property of food. The idea has been that if the calories going in (food) are less than the calories being used up (exercise), then you will lose weight. The theory is simple but as many women know, making it happen is much, much harder.

You might assume that if you lose weight on a crash diet you are burning off excess fat. But this can only be done slowly. Almost 25 percent of your weight loss will be water, bone, muscle and other lean tissue. As we have seen, the reason for this is that your body is programmed to hold onto fat and in times of what it considers to be famine will go as far as breaking down muscle and losing water in order to hold on to fat reserves. Although fad diets suggest that you can lose up to 10 pounds of weight in a week, it is very hard to lose more than 2 pounds of body fat.

What is the best way to lose weight?

Preparing for menopause involves some hard thinking about nutrition. You may well find that changing your eating habits to a healthier pattern will, over time, bring some of the elusive weight loss you have always longed for. If you lose weight gradually, it is more likely to stay off, so the best way is to follow the recommendations in Chapter 5. You need to find a way of eating that is enjoyable, nutritious, and also a way of life, not a diet you follow for a while and then abandon in favor of your old ways. I suggest that you eat little and often, basing your diet around good-quality complex carbohydrates, together with a small amount of healthy proteins, such as pulses (beans and related foods), fish and eggs plus plenty of fruit and vegetables. I know that this advice is not fashionable, but it is healthy and it works.

The truth about trendy diets

FOOD-COMBINING

You may have heard that following a food-combining diet can help you lose weight. This is an eating regime where protein and starch (carbohydrates) are eaten at separate meals, and is based on the belief that these foods need different enzymes to be digested effectively. It is claimed that if protein and starch are eaten together, two problems occur. First, undigested food is stored in the intestines where it ferments, leading to bloating and flatulence, and second, it is then stored as fat. Although there is no scientific proof for the theory, there are people who feel that food combining has helped their digestive problems. Weight loss is another matter, however, and critics often say that the reason it works is because it restricts food intake and helps you to become more aware of what you are eating.

HIGH-PROTEIN

This dietary regime is based on eating lots of meat and eggs but few carbohydrates and little fruit. It first became popular in the 1970s, but more recently it has been the latest craze to sweep the U.S., with a number of celebrities swearing by its ability to promote quick weight loss.

The diet sounds logical and it can have dramatic results, but in the long term, it is not only unhealthy but can be dangerous as well. Sweet and starchy foods make blood sugar levels rise sharply, increasing levels of insulin. More food is converted into fat and you begin to put on weight. The theory behind the high-protein diet is that by cutting out anything that prevents a surge of insulin, you will lose weight. It is certainly true that when the body is starved of carbohydrates, it raids its glycogen stores for energy, which makes it possible to lose a lot of weight very quickly. But the immediate weight loss is water, not fat, because 4 grams (0.14 ounce) of water cling to every gram of glycogen. Only when the glycogen stores are depleted does the body start to dissolve fat. A protein-only diet can cause an abnormal metabolic state called "ketosis," because there is not enough carbohydrate stored in the liver for the body to use. Ketones accumulate in the blood, causing side-effects such as bad breath (there is a fruity odor of acetone on the breath), poor concentration, mood swings and bad memory. These are not symptoms that you will want to experience, especially when you could already be suffering from them pre-menstrually. These same symptoms are evident in cases of starvation, and in diabetes mellitus. You could be having some of these symptoms as a result of menopause anyway, so you don't want to make the situation worse.

There are other damaging side-effects, too. One is an accumulation of nitrogen in the body. Nitrogen is a product of protein that is normally excreted through the urine. When the protein content of the diet is very high, excess nitrogen builds up and can damage the liver and kidneys. As if that were not enough, it is also known that the higher your protein intake, the greater your risk of losing bone density and therefore of osteoporosis. Protein causes an acidic reaction in the body and calcium acts as a neutralizer. When you eat too much protein, your reserves of calcium, which are contained in your bones and teeth, are summoned to correct the imbalance. It is estimated that for every extra 15 grams (0.5 ounce) of protein that you eat, you lose 100 grams (3 ounces) of calcium in your urine.

My advice is to avoid high-protein diets for two reasons. First and foremost, the body needs carbohydrates, and choosing the right kind – that is, complex, whole carbohydrates – will undoubtedly encourage weight loss as well as help to reduce menopausal problems by stabilizing blood sugar levels. Second, the price of cutting out carbohydrates altogether is simply too high. In the long run, your health could be compromised.

Which foods make you fat?

You may be surprised to hear that fat and thin people often eat roughly the same calories; it is the type of food they eat rather than the amount that makes the difference. Food can be converted into fat or energy by chemical reactions activated by enzymes, which are dependent upon vitamins and minerals. Your body can either store what you eat or convert it into the energy you need to do what your want with your life. But not all foods are easy to convert into energy, and these are the ones most likely to make you put on weight.

FAT

Because fat is high in calories, more and more women are buying low-fat and non-fat foods. Yes, 50–60 percent of calories in the average Western diet come from fats, and by cutting down, it is possible to lose weight. But it is saturated fats from animal foods such as milk, cheese, eggs, poultry and meat that need to be kept to a minimum. It is unhealthy and counterproductive to go on a virtually fat-free diet, which can result in joint stiffness, skin problems and vaginal dryness.

Certain fats are vital for good health, which is why they are called essential fats or essential fatty acids (EFAs). Your body cannot make essential fats, so the only source is your diet – nuts (almonds, pecans, brazils and so on), seeds (such as sesame, sunflower, pumpkin), oils (olive, sunflower, sesame), oily fish (tuna, mackerel, salmon) and vegetables. These unsaturated essential fats are a vital component of every human cell and your body needs them to insulate your nerve cells, keep your skin and arteries supple, balance your hormones and keep you warm. They have also been found to relieve benign breast disease and what is more, may actually help you lose weight because they increase metabolic rate and speed up the rate at which body fat is burned.

SUGAR

Sugar is empty calories. It has no nutritional value, so avoiding it is crucial if you want to lose weight. Every time you eat your body has a choice: it can either burn food as energy or store it as fat. Any food or drink that makes blood sugar fluctuate and insulin soar (see page 65) will change more of your food into fat and will stop your body breaking down previously stored fat. I see a lot of women who are restricting their calories, eating low-fat everything and taking good levels of exercise, yet not losing weight. That is because their bodies are turning food into fat instead of using it as energy.

Added sugar is not the only problem. Refined carbohydrates (which are stripped of fiber) are digested very quickly, so glucose enters the bloodstream too rapidly. Glucose is the fastest-acting carbohydrate because it needs no processing before it passes into the bloodstream and raises insulin very quickly. This sharp rise in blood glucose means that your body has to secrete more insulin to deal with it. The message to your body is to "store fat" – hence the weight gain.

You can work out the glucose level of the food you eat by referring to the glycemic index (GI), which measures how quickly or slowly a food releases glucose into the bloodstream. Pure glucose has a score of 100, and all foods are measured against this. The less refined a carbohydrate (for example, brown rice, whole grains and vegetables) the lower the GI, because the fiber in these foods slows down the release of sugars. Similarly, whole fruit has a lower GI than fruit juice, because fiber slows down the absorption of sugar.

The most important piece of information that has emerged from the GI is that contrary to the principles of food combining, it is actually beneficial to combine proteins and carbohydrates. The presence of protein in food (either animal or vegetable) actually lowers its glycemic index. So fish and rice (preferably brown) or rice and tofu are actually good combinations. Pulses, such as lentils, which naturally contain both protein and carbohydrate, have a low GI.

The simplest way to work out the glycemic rating of a food without resorting to the chart is to consider how refined it is. The more refined the food, the faster it is digested, and the bigger its impact on your insulin levels. Highly refined foods will make any menopausal symptoms worse, so go for unprocessed foods and base your diet around fiber-rich foods that have a lower GI, such as brown rice, because fiber slows down the release of sugars. Caffeine also triggers the fast release of insulin, so if you want to lose weight then eliminate tea, coffee and chocolate.

Once your taste buds are accustomed to this new way of eating, sugary foods will start to seem too sweet. In the meantime, try to resist artificial sweeteners. Aspartame, for example, is 180 times sweeter than sugar and it can lead to binge-eating and weight problems. Although women are often misled into believing that sweeteners like this can help to control weight, it has been found that people who use them regularly tend to gain weight, because sweeteners increase the appetite.[1]

The glycemic index of common foods

Sugars	serving	GI Score	Sugars	serving	GI Score
Glucose			Potatoes *(fried)*	4.3 oz.	75
powder	2 tablets	102	Sweet potatoes		
Honey	1 tbs.	58	*(boiled)* 1/2 cup		54
Sucrose *(sugar)*	1 tsp.	65			
			Grains and Cereals		GI Score
Fruit			Bagel	1 small	72
Apple	1 medium	38	Barley	1/2 cup	26
Apple juice	8 oz.	40	Basmati rice	1 cup	58
Banana	1 medium	62	Brown rice	1 cup	55
Cantaloupe	1/4 small	65	French baguette	1 oz.	95
Cherries	10 large	22	Muesli	2/3 cup	43
Grapefruit	1/2 medium	25	Oatmeal	1 cup	49
Grapes	3 oz.	46	White bread	1 slice	70
Kiwi fruit	1 medium	52	White rice	1 cup	72
Orange	1 medium	40	White spaghetti	1 cup	41
Orange juice	8 oz.	46	Whole grain		
Pear	1 medium	38	rye bread	1 slice	65
Pineapple			Whole grain		
(fresh)	4 oz.	66	spaghetti	1 cup	42
Plum	1 medium	39	Whole grain		
Raisins	1/4 cup	64	wheat bread	1 slice	69
Watermelon	1 cup	72			
			Pulses		
Vegetables			Baked beans	1/2 cup	48
Beets *(cooked)*	1/2 cup	64	Blackeyed peas	1/2 cup	42
Carrots *(boiled)*	1/2 cup	49	Butter beans	1/2 cup	31
Parsnips *(boiled)*		97	Chick peas		
Peas	1/2 cup	48	*(canned)*	1/2 cup	36
Potato chips	14 pieces	54	Haricot beans		31
Potatoes			Kidney beans	3 oz.	27
(baked)	1 medium	85	Lentils	4 oz.	29
Potatoes			Soy beans	1/2 cup	15
(boiled new)	4 oz.	70			

Extra help for weight loss

A number of chemical reactions are involved in turning glucose into energy rather than fat. These are controlled by enzymes, which are dependent on certain vitamins and minerals. If these are deficient, you will lack energy and feel low. So you can help yourself by making sure that you have a balanced intake.

• B vitamins help to supply cells with fuel ready for burning as energy. Vitamin B6 is especially important because it is necessary for the production of pancreatic enzymes that help efficient digestion.

• Chromium is a mineral that has been widely researched in connection with weight loss. It is needed for the metabolism of sugar – without it insulin is less effective in controlling blood sugar levels.[2] It helps to reduce hunger and cravings and to control fat and cholesterol in the blood. One study showed that people who took a chromium supplement over a 10-week period lost an average of 4.2 pounds of fat while those on a placebo (dummy tablet) lost only 0.4 pound.[3]

• Co-Enzyme Q10 is important for energy production. It is found in all the body's tissues and organs but reduces with age, which results in energy depletion. It has been used to help heart problems, high blood pressure, gum disease and immune problems and has also been shown to encourage weight loss. A study showed that people on a low-fat diet doubled their weight loss when taking Q10 compared to those who used diet alone.[4]

• *Garcinia cambogia*, a small tropical fruit whose rind is used in Thai and Indian cooking, contains hydroxy-citric acid (HCA), which encourages the conversion of carbohydrates into energy rather than fat. The HCA in the fruit seems to curb appetite, reduce food intake and inhibit the formation of fat and cholesterol.

• Vitamin C helps to lower cholesterol and is involved in the conversion of glucose to energy in the cells.

• Zinc is an important mineral in appetite control. A deficiency of zinc causes a loss of taste and smell, so that you crave stronger-tasting foods. Zinc also works with vitamin B6 to make the enzyme that digests food.

Medical reasons for weight gain

What can you do if you are eating well and taking exercise and still the weight does not shift? First of all, ask your doctor whether any medication you may be taking (such as oral steroids) could be causing weight gain (but do not stop the medication without discussing it with your doctor), or whether you could have a medical condition that is causing the problem, such as:

Underactive thyroid

If you answer "yes" to four or more of the following questions, ask your doctor to test your thyroid hormone level.

• Has your weight increased gradually over the past few months for no apparent reason?
• Do you often feel cold?
• Are you constipated?
• Do you feel depressed, forgetful or confused?
• Are you losing your hair or is it drier than it used to be?
• Have you noticed a lack of energy?
• Are you getting headaches?

The thyroid gland situated in your neck is like a thermostat that regulates your body temperature. It secretes two hormones, thyroxine and triiodothyronine, which control how quickly the body burns calories and uses energy. An underactive thyroid (hypothyroidism) is caused by one of two things: either your pituitary gland is not producing sufficient thyroid-stimulating hormones or the thyroid itself is not working properly.

The first thing you can do if you suspect that all is not well is to ask your doctor for a blood test to establish how efficiently your thyroid is functioning. If it detects an underactive thyroid, you will probably be prescribed a drug called thyroxine. This is usually well tolerated, although you should be monitored to ensure that you are taking the correct dose because side-effects can be a problem if it is given in excessively high doses.

Unfortunately mild problems may not be detected by this test. Someone with all the symptoms of an underactive thyroid may have normal blood levels because although the thyroid gland is producing enough hormones, the cells that are supposed to latch on to them are not picking them up.

This is where self-help comes in because you can test for low thyroid function simply by measuring your temperature. If it is too low, it may indicate that you have a sluggish metabolism caused by an underactive thyroid. Take your temperature first thing in the morning for three consecutive days, before getting up or having anything to eat or drink. If you are past menopause you can do this at any time of the month, but if you are still having periods, take your temperature on the second, third and fourth days of your cycle – in other words, start the day after your period begins. Because your body temperature rises after ovulation, you will not get a clear picture if you take it later in the cycle. Put the thermometer in your armpit and leave it until it bleeps. (If you are using a mercury thermometer, leave it for 10 minutes.) If your average temperature for the three days falls below 97.6ÞF (36.4ÞC), your thyroid may be underfunctioning.

NATURAL THYROID TREATMENTS

It is possible to manage mild thyroid problems by making simple changes to your diet. The two hormones produced by the thyroid gland (thyroxine and triidothyronine) are made from iodine and the amino acid tyrosine. If you have an underactive thyroid, it is important to avoid foods that interfere with the uptake of these nutrients and eat more of those that contain them.

Foods called goitrogens, which block the uptake of iodine, will make an underactive thyroid problem worse. They include turnips, cabbage, peanuts, soy, pine nuts and millet. These foods only seem to be a problem when they are raw and eaten excessively, so make sure they are cooked well and eat them in moderation.

Whenever possible, opt for naturally rich sources of iodine such as seafoods, especially saltwater fish, and seaweeds such as kelp. Seaweed contains the trace minerals zinc, manganese, chromium, selenium and cobalt and the macro minerals calcium, magnesium, iron, as well as iodine. Scientific studies show that it can also have anti-cancer benefits[5] and can reduce cholesterol and improve fat metabolism.[6]

Supplements can also optimize thyroid gland function, but as too much iodine can actually make an underactive thyroid condition worse, I recommend seeing a qualified practitioner for help. One useful mineral is selenium, which helps the thyroid hormones to function properly. Low levels have been linked to underactive thyroid problems,[7] but taking 100 micrograms per day should restore the balance.

Herbalists have traditionally used a type of seaweed called bladderwrack (*Fucus vesiculosus*) to boost a sluggish thyroid. This is normally taken as a tablet, but if you are lucky enough to be able to buy it fresh or dried, you can make an infusion by pouring a cup of boiling water onto 2 to 3 teaspoons of dried bladderwrack and leaving it for 10 minutes. This infusion can be drunk three times a day.

Food allergy

Although some food allergies are sudden and life-threatening, others take longer to make an impact. A classic Type-A allergy to an allergen such as peanuts causes a severe reaction immediately, but a Type-B delayed allergy (sometimes called food intolerance) has an effect between one hour and four days after contact with the allergen.

Common Type-B allergens include dairy products, eggs, wheat and sugar, which can cause symptoms such as weight gain, bloating, water retention, fatigue, aching joints and headaches. Despite the damaging effect of these foods, they often become mildly addictive and you can feel compelled to eat them. If you suspect you may have a Type-B allergy, a good question to ask is, "What food or drink would you find it hard to give up?"

You can find out if your suspicions are correct by having a blood test that analyzes 217 different foods and food additives by measuring the release of the chemicals responsible for your symptoms. Once you know the foods that are causing the problems, you can avoid them for a short period of time and reduce your sensitivity. As long as your allergy is Type B rather than Type A (which can be fatal) these foods do not have to avoided indefinitely. The aim is to exclude them from your diet for a time, allowing you to strengthen and correct any digestive problems so that eventually you can eat them in moderation.

Mood-boosting food

Food and mood go together, which is why you may cheer yourself up with a chocolate bar when you feel down. And with reason, because there are substances in chocolate that do indeed impart a "feel-good" factor.

Chocolate is just one of the foods that can trigger all kinds of important changes in brain chemistry. What you eat and drink can determine whether you feel happy or depressed, give comfort and ward off boredom. These powerful brain chemicals also affect appetite and the ability to control it, and you may eat more when you feel sad or lonely. So being aware of what controls your appetite and eating patterns is crucial if you want to lose weight and establish a healthy diet.

Understanding the different biochemical reactions of food on your mood means that you can use what you eat to your advantage – with one proviso. A wide, varied diet is vital, because the balance of the brain chemicals can be disturbed by nutritional deficiencies and by poor diet. The more restricted your choice of foods, the harder it is for your body to help the brain to maintain this important balance.

That said, it is relatively simple to improve your mood by choosing the right foods. If you want to feel more alert, for example, make sure you eat enough protein. Protein contains an amino acid called tyrosine, which manufactures the brain chemicals norepinephrine (noradrenaline) and dopamine that help to focus your mind.

If you need to de-stress, on the other hand, steer clear of too much protein and opt for calming carbohydrates instead. Complex carbohydrates such as rice and oats increase the levels of serotonin, which controls appetite and boosts your mood, making you feel happier and more relaxed. They do this by acting on an amino acid called tryptophan that stimulates the production of serotonin, and by helping the body to release insulin. Insulin mops up the other amino acids in the system, which increases the effect of tryptophan and so raises levels of feel-good serotonin. The opposite happens when you eat a protein-rich meal or snack. This releases a number of amino acids that compete with each other to get into the brain so tryptophan cannot dominate.

Eating little and often and keeping your blood sugar in balance are important ways to stabilize serotonin too. If you eat too little, your serotonin level, which regulates mood and appetite, will fall. You may start to feel more anxious and begin to overeat. In contrast, a regular intake of complex carbohydrates means you can control your moods and your appetite, without feeling deprived or hungry.

Other ways of controlling your appetite include eating more slowly. The chemical cholecystokinin (CCK) is released as food enters the stomach. It tells the digestion to slow down and then gives the message to the brain that you are "full" so your appetite naturally decreases. The message normally takes about 20 minutes to get through, so you need to give your brain, and your appetite, time to receive the signal that you have eaten enough.

Exercise can also help. Although the appetite-boosting brain chemical neuropeptide Y increases when you exercise, it makes you want to eat complex carbohydrates. These release serotonin, which makes you feel good and keeps your appetite under control.

Six ways to fight food cravings

1. Be aware of your food triggers
Feeling low can easily lead to comfort-eating. Do you eat differently when you feel sad, lonely or bored? If so, look at what you could substitute for food. Mixing with other people can help to shift the emphasis away from yourself, so it might be worth finding a new hobby, doing voluntary work or joining an evening class.

Eating from habit is another common problem. You may find yourself munching almost automatically if you link food to certain activities such as watching TV. One woman who consulted me had gotten into the habit of coming home from work and almost unconsciously going to the fridge. Awareness of what you are doing and when is the key. Stop, think, and ask yourself, "Do I really need to eat this now? Will I be happy with the way I feel after I have eaten it?"

2. Exercise
Going for a brisk walk or a swim can help to ward off a craving. Exercise releases chemicals in the brain that make you feel good, so that you no longer need food to do that for you.

3. Eat plenty of complex carbohydrates
You will be amazed at how much filling and satisfying food you can eat and still lose weight. That is because starchy foods, such as rice, millet, whole wheat, rye, oats and barley, keep your blood sugar in balance, so your body automatically stops craving a quick fix. Complex carbohydrates work slowly, providing sustained levels of energy and helping you to feel satisfied for longer. They burn like coal, building up heat slowly and releasing warmth over a long period of time. Eating refined starch and sugar, on the other hand, is like setting fire to a newspaper, which gives a quick burst of heat and then goes out!

4. Distract yourself
If you know that certain situations make you want certain foods, either avoid the situation or else prepare a healthy alternative to curb your appetite. Cravings will disappear if you don't satisfy them, so do something to occupy your hands, read or make a phone call, and see what you feel like after that.

5. Eat little and often
Do not go for more than three hours during the day without food. If you do, your blood sugar level will drop and your body will automatically crave something sweet. If you wait a long while between meals you may actually end

up eating more because long gaps raise levels of the brain chemical neuropeptide-Y, which increases hunger and may even cause binging. What is more, your body will go into famine-mode and slow your metabolism down, so you can end up putting on more weight than you otherwise would. The answer is to have snacks of complex carbohydrates between meals to keep your blood sugar even.

6. Don't deny yourself

If you vow never to eat chocolate again, you are likely to fail. Be realistic; you can't be sensible all the time. If you keep denying yourself, when you eventually crack you will probably end up eating far more than if you had allowed yourself an occasional indulgence. If your nutrition is basically good, then relax and enjoy yourself. If a friend fancies an ice cream or chocolate bar, have one too. But buy the best quality you can and be aware of the taste while you eat it.

If you follow the recommendations in Chapter 5 and eat little and often, you will find that cravings just disappear. One woman who came to my clinic complained that in the week before her period, she would sit and eat boxes of chocolates during the afternoon. She just couldn't stop herself. I explained about blood sugar swings and cravings, and she agreed to eat little and often during her next cycle, with more emphasis on complex carbohydrates. She wasn't convinced it would be effective and kept saying, "This isn't going to work." Instead of arguing, I replied "What have you got to lose, except the binges?"

When I saw her a month later, she was amazed to find that the cravings had gone. But what surprised her most was the way they had gone. She hadn't needed to use will power at all. Because her body didn't need chocolate, it didn't ask her for it, and she had gone through the whole cycle without giving it a thought. When she went out for dinner and was offered an after-dinner mint, her reaction was, "Well, I can take this or leave it." And she left it.

What controls your appetite?

Among the brain chemicals (neurotransmitters) that send signals to the brain cells (neurons) telling them to act, there are several that control your appetite.

These brain chemicals increase your intake of food:
• endorphins – give a "natural buzz," a sense of euphoria

continued

- norepinephrine (noradrenaline) – makes you feel alert and energetic
- neuropeptide Y – released during exercise, gives you an appetite for carbohydrates.

These decrease your appetite:
- cholecystokinin (CCK) – tells the brain you are full so your appetite decreases
- serotonin – makes you feel calm and sleepy and can lift depression
- corticotropin releasing factor – suppresses appetite.

Feel better all day

Look at your own daily pattern and work out the best meals (and meal-times) for you, using the following guide.

Breakfast
A breakfast based on carbohydrates such as oatmeal has a positive mood-enhancing effect. Don't skip breakfast, even if you find that eating first thing makes you feel hungry all day. If this is the case, eat a high-protein breakfast, such as scrambled eggs with a slice of whole grain or rye bread.

Lunch
Eating a high-carbohydrate meal, such as a baked potato, at midday can make you feel relaxed and sleepy. The body naturally has a "post-lunch dip" so you may find it difficult to keep your eyes open. Other countries are aware of this and have a siesta, but a 9-to-5 working day forces you to battle your way through the afternoon. To feel alert and focused, eat a higher protein meal for lunch such as a tuna salad with a small portion of rice or a rye cracker. However, if you crave sweets and chocolates mid-afternoon, you need to eat complex carbohydrates for lunch and also as an afternoon snack.

Dinner
If you find you turn to alcohol to help you relax in the evening, have a high carbohydrate evening meal such as brown rice and tofu stir-fry.

CHAPTER 12

The Benefits of Exercise and Sex at Menopause

It is impossible to exaggerate the benefits of regular exercise. It has a direct impact on the way you feel and look, on your bone strength, your heart function and your hormones, and the older you get, the more important it is for your health. Regular exercise appears to be linked to a lower risk of breast cancer and a higher tolerance of stress and is absolutely vital for any woman who wants to keep a youthful figure, glowing skin and a general zest for life.

Exercise has an important role to play during menopause, although quite how important we may never know. The vast majority of medical research is devoted to finding "cures" for "symptoms." The pharmaceutical industry wants products to sell. It is not terribly interested in publicizing the fact that exercise may prevent or relieve menopausal symptoms, which is why the benefits of exercise are not examined more closely or promoted more aggressively.

Exercise can help ...

... YOUR EMOTIONS

When you exercise, the brain releases chemicals called endorphins that help you feel happier, calmer and more alert. Exercise has been shown to have a dramatic and positive effect on people suffering from depression, stress, anxiety and insomnia, and is now often recommended as part of a treatment program for these problems.

... YOUR BONES

The impact of exercise on bone has been dramatically illustrated by research carried out on the bone density of professional tennis players. In the racket-holding arm, which does most of the work, bone density is over a third greater than it is in the other arm. Any activity that makes a demand on your bones helps to maintain bone density and prevent osteoporosis. This is called weight-bearing exercise and it includes brisk walking, running, badminton, stair climbing and aerobics, as well as tennis. It doesn't matter which one you do, the important thing is to do it, because women who allow themselves to become inactive are at risk of fractures in later life. If you are sedentary and make no demands on your bones, you risk compromising your bone health.

Bodily functions are very logical. Astronauts lose bone density in the weightlessness of space where there is no pressure on their bones, and the same principle applies to everyone else. If you tell your body that you need strong bones, your bone density will be maintained or increased. The process is simple. When it detects that the bones are under stress, your body creates more bone by drawing bone-building cells called osteoblasts to the areas where they are needed. It is another case of "use it or lose it."

One word of caution. While several studies have shown that weight-bearing exercise helps women to maintain or increase their bone density through and beyond menopause, you need to be careful not to put too much strain on your joints. A study by researchers from St. Thomas's Hospital London in the *Journal of Arthritis and Rheumatism* compared former athletes with a group of ordinary women, all with an average age of 52. Although the bones of the former athletes were 15 percent stronger than those of the others, they were also more likely to show signs of wear and tear in the joints (osteoarthritis). Clearly the answer is to find forms of exercise that increase demands on the bones but that also avoid too much pressure on joints. The recommendations of the St. Thomas's team were to do an hour's intensive weight-bearing exercise a week, or two hours of walking. They also felt that short bursts of activity, such as running for 10 minutes, could be beneficial as long as they took place every day.

... YOUR AGILITY

Exercise does more than improve the strength of your bones; it also keeps your reflexes sharp and improves coordination. As you get older, your range of movement becomes limited unless you make the effort to maintain it. Many fractures are caused by falling, or missing a step. If you keep yourself flexible and have good reflexes and coordination, you may save yourself from falling. Exercise also helps to build up the muscles, and strong muscles act as the first line of defense when you have an accident, shielding your bones from impact.

... YOUR APPETITE

Besides releasing feel-good endorphins, exercise stimulates several other brain chemicals. Corticotropin Releasing Factor (CRF) suppresses appetite so that you don't want to stuff yourself with food after aerobics although you have used up plenty of calories. Even when this effect wears off, the kind of food your body demands is very different. Another brain chemical, neuropeptide Y, also released when you exercise, increases your need for carbohydrates, the body's prime source of energy, by telling your body what kind of fuel it needs. Although energy is also supplied by fats and to a lesser degree protein, the main source should be starchy foods, such as rice, wheat, rye and oats. So exercise, which uses up energy, releases brain chemicals that make you eat more of the foods that give you more energy. It's a very clever system that demonstrates yet again how given the chance, your body will find the right balance.

... YOUR HEART

Exercise improves the circulation and seems to lower LDL (bad) cholesterol while increasing HDL (good) cholesterol. It can also help to reduce blood pressure, one of the main risk factors for heart disease. Exercise allows the blood to keep circulating freely instead of becoming obstructed, so it can do a lot to help varicose veins. "Tired" or "heavy" legs respond well to regular walking or jogging.

... YOUR WEIGHT

Exercise helps fat burn more efficiently, boosting your metabolism so that you use up calories faster, even after you stop exercising. This is particularly important if you are on a diet, because your metabolism tries to slow down when you reduce the amount of food you eat. You can increase the fat-burning effect still more by combining aerobic activity with weight- or resistance-training, which builds muscle. Muscle requires more feeding than other tissue to survive because it is more metabolically active, so if you have a bit more muscle, you use up more calories. One pound of muscle can burn 35–50 calories a day, whereas a pound of fat burns only two or three.

The housework workout

How many calories do you burn off doing everyday activities? This is how many you use in 20 minutes.

Activity	Calories burned
Ironing	20
Housework	60
Mowing the lawn	60
Digging	100
Walking upstairs	120
Running upstairs	200

... YOUR HORMONES

Exercise helps to keep your adrenal glands healthy, which is crucial at menopause since they become your main source of estrogen.

The adrenal glands and stress hormones

The adrenal glands perch on top of your kidneys. They consist of two parts – the medulla, which secretes the stress hormones adrenaline and noradrenaline (norepinephrine), and the cortex, which produces three kinds of hormones, including the sex hormones. As your ovaries slow down, your adrenal glands take over, producing not only estrone (a form of estrogen) but also male hormones (androgens), which give you drive and zest.

To maximize the release of these sex hormones, you need to make sure that the adrenals do not concentrate all their efforts on producing stress hormones. Adrenaline and noradrenaline are designed to be released in a "fight or flight" situation. At times of danger, you need either to run or to defend yourself. Your body's response is immediate and dramatic. Your liver releases stored sugar into the bloodstream to supply instant energy. Blood is taken away from the skin and moved into muscles and internal organs. Your heart speeds up and your arteries tighten, raising your blood pressure so blood is moved to where it is needed most. Your digestion shuts down because your energy is needed elsewhere. At the same time your blood thickens, ready to clot in case you are injured.

All this happens very fast and should stop as soon as you are out of danger, giving the adrenals time to recuperate. But modern life creates different kinds of stresses that affect the body in the same way as a threat to your life. Say you are stuck in a traffic jam, late for an appointment, getting more and more stressed and eating your lunch at the same time. All the stress responses kick into play with the important difference that you cannot fight or flee: in a traffic jam all you can do is to sit there and seethe. All this is made worse by the fact that you could be in that traffic jam for a long time, so the effect is not going to be short-lived. So what happens? Your digestion has shut down, although you are trying to eat, so you could get indigestion or not absorb the nutrients from your food properly. Your blood starts to clot more rapidly – and what will that do to your risk of heart attack and strokes?

Many people today are under so much stress that the adrenal glands are in constant demand and may become exhausted. It is not just the odd traffic jam. It is the pressure of work, the demands of family, money worries... the list goes on. Every day there are many occasions when the

continued

body is put on a biochemical "red alert." If the body has no physical outlet for all this inactive stress, it reacts in other ways and you suffer from symptoms such as backache, shoulder pain, tension headaches, digestive problems, ulcers and high blood pressure. Exercise gives your body the proper physical outlet for all that stress, enabling your hormone systems to get back in balance.

... YOUR DIGESTION

Regular activity helps to keep your bowels working efficiently, so you eliminate the waste products your body doesn't need. Exercise is a prime treatment for constipation and also helps the body to keep your blood sugar in balance, so that you are in more control of your weight and your moods.

... YOUR MIND

Exercise can have a positive effect on brain function. Growing evidence that an inactive lifestyle may be linked to brain degeneration indicates that by keeping active, you may be able to retain your brain power as you grow older and reduce the risk of developing of Alzheimer's disease. Regular exercise has also been shown to help with insomnia because moderate exercise performed at any time of day except just before bed can improve sleep quality.

... YOUR LOVE LIFE

Energy and vitality help you to get the best out of life, not least because they increase your interest in sex. You may feel that you are just too tired to have sex, but if you make an effort to exercise, your libido will wake up. You know how your interest in sex can perk up when you are on vacation. There are no pressures, you are more relaxed, and you also have more energy. Why wait for this to happen maybe once a year? Get fit and active, and enjoy making love.

Sexual exercise

Some forms of exercise have specific benefits for your love life. Exercises such as swimming and cycling, which promote the blood supply to the vaginal area, can help with vaginal dryness. Special exercises developed by Dr. Arnold Kegel in the 1940s not only counteract vaginal dryness by stimulating the blood supply but also make sex more enjoyable by increasing the strength of your vaginal sensations. Sometimes called pelvic floor exercises, they strengthen the muscles in the pelvic area, helping to prevent stress incontinence (when you "leak" small amounts of urine when you laugh, sneeze or run).

There are two groups of muscles that need to be worked and two types of exercises to work them. First of all, slowly raise your pelvic floor by contracting the muscles. Hold for a count of five and then gently let it down again. Work at this several times a day until you can hold for a count of 15. You may find that you lose control partway through the count. Start again, making sure that you can feel the muscles being released as you "let down" your pelvic floor. The second type of exercise involves quickly tightening and releasing the muscles in the pelvic floor. As fast as you can, tighten and then release the muscles. Do this about 30 times, then take a break.

Each session should comprise two sets of slow exercises and two sets of fast, with a minute's break in between. Some women find it easier to practice these exercises while sitting on a kitchen chair because you can actually feel the muscles as they rise and fall against the seat, but in the beginning it may help to perform them lying down, to reduce the pressure of gravity. If you find it difficult to locate the correct muscles, go to the bathroom and try to stop your urine flow in midstream. You shouldn't do this regularly, however, because it can push urine back up into the bladder, leading to infections and bladder weakness.

I found that these exercises helped me significantly. After the birth of my third child, who was a fairly large 9 pounds 9 ounces, I suspected I had a vaginal prolapse. It seemed to get better but a couple of years later I had the dragging feeling again, and consulted my doctor. He confirmed that I had a slight prolapse and said I should come back for treatment when it got worse. I found this rather unhelpful. My objective was to stop it from getting worse, in case it got to the point where I might have to have a hysterectomy. So deciding to practice what I preach, I looked for some alternatives. I went to see an acupuncturist, took herbs, and did Kegel exercises. Seventeen years later I still feel fine. It could be argued that maybe the herbs would have worked on their own, or perhaps it was the acupuncture, and that it had nothing to do with the exercises. Maybe. Whether it was one of those or a combination of all three, it worked.

Pelvic tilt and bow

These exercises should improve circulation in the pelvic area and enhance your sex life.

The pelvic tilt
Lie on your back with your knees bent. Slowly tilt and curl your pelvis. Hold for 20 seconds and then let go. Continue for five minutes.

continued

> *The bow*
> Standing with your hands on your hips, breathe deeply and then bend
> your knees. Suck in your stomach and arch your back. Hold for 20
> seconds and then let go. Repeat for five minutes.

How old is your body?

Biological age can differ from chronological age. The difference, scientists
believe, is caused by a number of things that include your genetic inheritance
and lifestyle factors, such as diet, smoking, drinking and exercise.

This test, reproduced by kind permission of the London *Daily Mail* from
an article by Andrew Willson (April 1995), can give an approximate indication
of your biological age. Circle the number after each of your answers and add
them up to give a total score.

1. *Do you or have you ever smoked?*

No, never	1
Once or twice	3
A few a day	4
A packet a day	5

2. *Do you drink? (1 unit is a glass of wine or $1\frac{1}{42}$ pint of beer or 1 measure of hard liquor)*

No, never	3
1–2 units a day	1
3–4 units a day	4
More than this	5

3. *How many servings of high-fat foods (fried food, dairy products, etc.) do you have a day?*

None	1
Two or three	3
Three to six	4
More than this	5

4. *How often to you eat red meat?*

Never	1
Three to five times a week	4
More than this	5

5. *How often do you eat fish?*

Never	5
Once a week	3
Twice a week	2
Three or more	1

6. *How many servings of pieces of fruit and vegetables do you eat each day?*

None	5
One or two	3
Three or four	2
Five or more	1

7. *Do you sunbathe or work outdoors without adequate protection from the sun's rays?*

Yes, all the time	5
Once or twice a year	4
Never	1

8. *With your thumb and forefinger, pinch a piece of skin on the back of your hand and hold in this position for five seconds. Release and then count how many seconds it takes for the skin to resume its original position.*

Age 40s–50s		*Age 60+*	
One second	1	Five or less seconds	1
Two seconds	2	Six to ten seconds	2
Three or four seconds	3	Eleven to sixteen seconds	3
Five to ten seconds	4	Sixteen to twenty seconds	4
More than ten seconds	5	More than twenty-one seconds	5

9. *Examine one of your fingernails under a bright light. Turn it slowly so you can see the texture of the nail.*

	Age 40+	*Age 50+*	*Age 60+*
No ridging or discoloration	1	1	1
Slight ridging	1	1	1
Noticeable ridging	5	3	3
Very noticeable ridging	5	3	3
Severe and extreme ridging	5	5	5

10. How many hours of exercise do you do a week?

	Age 40s–50s	*Age 60+*
None	4	3

One	2	2
More than one	1	1

11. *Sit on the floor, extend your right leg straight in front of you, and place the heel of your left foot against your right thigh. Then stretch your right arm as far as it will go toward your toes. How far can you stretch?*

	Age 40s–50s	Age 60+
Your wrist on your toes	1	1
Your fingertips on your toes	2	1
Your fingers on your ankle	3	2
Your fingers on your sock line	4	3

12. *Sit on a bottom step with your legs stretched straight out in front of you, with your heels on the ground, and your toes pointing upwards. Move your body so that your hands rest on the top of the stair and gently ease yourself down, bending your elbows until they are at 90 degrees. Now try to push yourself back up.*
How many of these can you do easily?

Age 40s		Age 50s		Age 60+	
Seven+ lifts	1	Six+ lifts	1	Five+ lifts	1
Six	3	Five	3	Four	3
Five or fewer	5	Four or fewer	5	Three or fewer	5

13. *For this test you will need an 8-inch-high step or box and a wristwatch with a second hand. Step up with your left foot, then your right, then step back down with your left and back down with your right. Do 20 complete steps per minute and continue for 3 minutes. After the 3 minutes are up, wait 15 seconds and then take your pulse (see page 206), count for 15 seconds, multiply this by four to get the total number of beats per minute and write this down. Then check your figure against your age group.*

Age 40s		Age 50+	
100 beats per minute	1	100 beats per minute	1
145 beats per minute	3	150 beats per minute	3
175 beats per minute	5	175 beats per minute	5

14. *How would you rate your general outlook on life?*

You can't bear to get out of bed in the morning	5
Generally pessimistic	4
Content	3
You try to look on the bright side	2
You see each day as a fresh challenge	1

15. *How do you react in stressful situations?*

Panic and fall to pieces	5
Get angry and lose your temper	4
Take a couple of deep breaths but still don't know how to deal with the problem	3
Calmly assess the situation and try to solve it	2
Thrive on stress and use it positively	1

How DID YOU SCORE?

Up to 15

You could be between five and 10 years younger than your chronological age. Carry on with your healthy diet and lifestyle and continue exercising.

Between 16 and 31

You could be between two and five years younger than your actual age, depending on whether you are closer to the higher or lower score. If you want to improve your score, then look at those areas where you scored two or above and see what changes you can make.

From 32 to 47

If you scored at the lower end of this category the test indicates that you are biologically a couple of years younger than your chronological age. If you are near the score of 47, your chronological and biological ages are almost the same. Look at the questions where you circled three or above and see what changes you can make.

Between 48 and 63

Scoring nearing the 48 mark means that your body is likely to be a few years older than average for your age. If your score is nearer 63, then you could be up to five years older than your chronological age. Follow the recommendations in this book and make some definite changes.

Between 64 and 79

You are getting old before your time. A score near 64 suggests you may be at least five years older than your chronological age whereas a score nearer 79 means you could be up to 10 years older. Look at your lifestyle. It is never too late to change and the body is very resilient.

Exercise for beginners

A few generations ago, exercise was part of everyday life. Both my father and mother would walk a few miles to work and back each day. After my sister and I were born, my mother would make her daily shopping trip on foot, and carry her purchases home. Washing was done weekly by hand and involved a lot of scrubbing and wringing out of clothes, strengthening the back and the wrists. Every job required effort and was physically demanding. What do I do? I put the family's clothes in the washing machine, turn it on and then take the clothes out. I drive the car to the supermarket once a week to pick up the shopping. To keep myself active, I need to make exercise a conscious part of my life, so I deliberately choose to walk upstairs instead of taking the elevator, I walk up escalators, I run up the stairs at home, I park the car farther away than I need to and walk, except when doing the weekly shopping! No one would want to go back to the days when household chores required so much hard physical effort, but it is essential to find some way of making up for this lack of everyday exercise.

Since regular exercise is more beneficial than an occasional burst of activity, you need to find something you enjoy so that you are motivated enough to want to do it regularly. You also need an exercise routine that fits in with your family, your lifestyle and your finances. Some women prefer to exercise on their own, others need the motivation of a group or a friend to keep them going. Do whatever you need to keep active and fit.

If you are not used to exercise, take things slowly at first and build up your stamina gradually. A balanced approach is important, especially at menopause, so don't overdo it. When estrogen production in the ovaries winds down, some body fat is necessary because estrogen is still made by the fat cells. Too much exercise can cause a change in the body-fat ratio and stop your periods (amenorrhea) or in the case of very young athletes, prevent them from starting. This is the result of hormonal imbalance and carries the risk of reduced bone mineral density later on in life. Extreme exercise, such as running or going to the gym every day or training for a particular event, can put the body under more stress than the exercise relieves. Nutritional demands increase and excessive sweating can cause the loss of vital minerals such as zinc, potassium and sodium. Of course, this is not a problem for most people. But some women become hooked on exercise – often women who have had eating problems when they were younger.

If moderation is important, so is variety. You need weight-bearing exercise for your bones, aerobic exercise for your heart and circulation, and some kind of stretching exercise to keep you flexible and poised. My time is very limited so I choose from a range of exercises that give me all-around benefits. Some I can do at home and some I need to plan. I mix walking and running up the stairs with yoga, exercises from a video and visits to my local gym. This way I get the different kinds of exercise my body needs.

Start with 30 minutes of exercise once a week and gradually build up to one hour, three times per week, varying the type of exercise. Whatever you do, be sure to warm up properly by doing some stretching exercises, to reduce the risk of injury to your muscles and joints, and stretch again when you have finished. Some research has suggested that stretching does not prevent as many injuries as was thought, but even if the stretching stops just one injury, it is worth it. If you join an exercise class make sure the instructor is properly trained and that he or she teaches you to do the exercises in the right way. It is all too easy to damage your back by pulling on the wrong muscles.

If you prefer to exercise on your own, try:

WALKING

If you have not exercised for years, brisk walking is a good way to start because there is little chance of injury. It has a number of other advantages. It can be fitted in at any time and does not require special equipment or clothing. It costs virtually nothing – indeed, it can save you money on gasoline and parking fees. It is an excellent weight-bearing exercise that helps protect your bones, and it frees the mind, so your imagination gets a workout too.

STRETCHING

Many years ago I was taught a series of yoga movements called the Sun Salutation, and they have stayed with me ever since. They are intended to be used at the start the day but I often do them at other times. I particularly like this sequence because it offers a variety of movements with a definite start and finish. It is quick and easy to do and you can vary the speed to suit yourself. The benefits are many, including improved posture, deep breathing, spine stretching, increased flexibility, better circulation and relaxation. Strictly speaking the Sun Salutation sequence is those movements numbered 1-4 and back again, as illustrated opposite, but I do the sequence twice to exercise both sides of the body (illustrations 1-12). Depending on the time available you can repeat it any number of times.

SUN SALUTATION

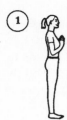

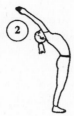

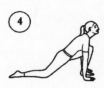

1 Stand up straight, shoulders back, feet together, arms hanging loosely at your sides. Breathe deeply and exhale as you bring your hands together in front of you.

2 Inhale and stretch your arms out over your head. Roll your hips forward and arch back from the waist, pushing your head back.

3 Exhale and slowly bend forward from the waist, placing your hands flat on the ground on either side of your feet, so that your fingers and toes form a straight line.

4 Inhale and, keeping your hands and feet in the same position, stretch your right leg back and drop your right knee to the ground.

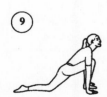

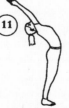

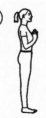

5 Holding your breath, take your left leg back. Straighten both legs and hold your body in a straight diagonal.

6 Exhale, bend your knees and place your knees, chest and forehead on the ground, raising your buttocks. Keep your elbows tucked in close to your body.

7 Inhale, slide your hips forward, point your toes back and arch your head and chest up and back. Keep your elbows bent and close to your sides.

8 Exhale, keep your hands in the same place, straighten your arms and lift your hips as high as possible while placing your feet flat on the floor.

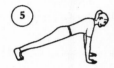

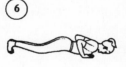

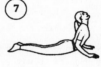

9 Inhale and, keeping your hands in the same place, drop your hips and stretch your left leg back. Drop your left knee to the ground, keeping your arms straight.

10 Exhale, bring your left foot forward and lift your hips up. Keep your hands on the ground and slide them towards you so that they are either side of your feet, with your toes and fingers aligned.

11 Inhale and stretch your arms out over your head. Roll your hips forwards and arch back from the waist, pushing your head back.

12 Stand up straight, shoulders back, feet together, arms hanging loosely at your sides. Exhale as you bring your hands together in front of you.

SWIMMING

Although it is not weight-bearing and will not strengthen your bones, swimming is a marvelous way to increase stamina, improve the functioning of your heart and lungs and give you a good stretch. Another option is aqua aerobics, which provides excellent cardiovascular exercise and muscle-toning without putting pressure on your joints. An additional bonus if you are on the plump side is that you will be more adept at water-based exercise than thinner women, whose lack of body fat makes it harder for them to float.

What's right for you?	
Exercise	*How it helps*
Brisk walking	Good weight-bearing exercise for the bones. Can be fitted in easily with your lifestyle. Healthy exercise for the heart, muscles and lungs.
Jogging/running	Good weight-bearing exercise for the bones. Can be fitted in at any time. Helps to release euphoria-linked endorphins and to lower cholesterol and prevent heart disease. Be careful of your joints if you are running on concrete: buy well-cushioned training shoes. And try not to run in a traffic-polluted area.
Rebounding	Uses a small trampoline at home, so you can do this exercise at any time. Gentle on the joints and a good weight-bearing exercise. Also good for the heart, lungs and circulation. There are books and videos available on this.
Racquet sports	Good weight-bearing activity. A sociable exercise that can be more motivating. Be sure that your racquet arm is not put under too much strain.
Swimming	Good aerobic activity for the heart and lungs. Easy on the joints but not weight-bearing. Osteopaths are concerned about the effect on the neck and back from the head being kept out of the water, so try to swim with your whole body in one line.

Dancing	A sociable, fun activity. Good for weight-bearing and also excellent for coordination that can prevent accidents at menopause.
Yoga	A good, all-around activity. Improves flexibility, suppleness and breathing. Excellent for the mind and body as it can help to reduce stress and give you tools to keep you calm
Cycling	A good exercise that can be done on an exercise bike or as a social activity. Excellent for muscle tone and strengthening, as well as pumping blood to the vaginal area.
Aerobic exercises	These are energetic movements performed to music. Good for the bones, heart and circulation. You can join a class which makes it more social, especially if you go with a friend. You can also use a video at home. Take things gradually at first and find the right level for yourself.
T'ai chi/qi gong	These are like moving meditations, which have mental as well as physical benefits. They need to be taught by an experienced practitioner and can then be practiced on your own. In China, the workforce of a company will perform these en masse before the start of a working day.
Alexander technique	This is not an exercise but a way of helping you to keep your posture as nature intended. Only the minimum effort is needed to produce a movement. As menopause takes place, there is the possibility of kyphosis (dowager's hump), so any help with your posture will be an advantage.

Exercise for the breasts

Although there are no muscles in your breasts, toning the pectoral muscles in your chest can help them to support their weight better and maintain their shape.

continued

• Stand two feet away from a wall and place your hands flat against it, one foot wider than your shoulders. Breathe in, bend your elbows, and lean towards the wall. Try to touch the wall with your nose, keeping your back flat and your legs straight as if you were doing a vertical press-up. Hold for a few seconds, then press away and repeat five times.

• Bend your elbows and press your palms together as if in a prayer position but with your elbows sticking out. Press your palms together as firmly as possible. Hold for a few seconds and then relax. Repeat five times.

Instant fitness check

You can find out how fit you are by measuring your pulse rate. Do this before you start and during exercise too, as a fast pulse rate will let you know that you are overdoing it. The less fit you are, the faster your pulse will be, because the heart has to work harder to pump blood around your body.

Your maximum pulse rate is 220, minus your age in years. So if you are 45, your maximum pulse rate will be 220-45 = 175.

To take your pulse at any given time, find the pulse in your wrist by placing three fingertips on the bone running down from your thumb. Move your fingers inward until you feel the beat. Count the number of beats for 30 seconds and double that figure to get your pulse rate per minute.

When you are exercising, check your pulse rate after three to four minutes. If you are unfit, you should aim for a pulse rate of 60 percent of your maximum, but if you are fit this can rise to 80 percent.

To check that you are exercising at the right level, look at the table below, which shows where your pulse rate should be after three to four minutes of exercise.

Age	Pulse rate (unfit)	Pulse rate (fit)
40	108	144
45	105	145
50	99	132
55	96	128

Sex is good for you

Sex not only feels good, it does you good. It releases brain chemicals known as endorphins that make you feel content and happy with the world. It stimulates the hormones, releases tension, helps to boost the immune system and can even relieve headaches. A massive research project involving 55,000 people conducted by the Institute for Advanced Study of Human Sexuality in San Francisco found that people who had a satisfying sex life were physically healthier and more relaxed than those who were not as fulfilled. Ted McIlvenna, President of the Institute, was even quoted as saying, "Sex is perhaps the best preventive and healing medicine there is." That may be a bit of an exaggeration but it makes the point that sex is important for a balanced, healthy life.

Perking up the libido is one of the supposed benefits of taking hormone replacement therapy. But there is no real evidence that tinkering with hormone levels has any effect on a woman's sexuality at all. What may undermine it, however, is the notion that menopause is some kind of crisis, that when the biological clock starts to chime a woman inevitably becomes less attractive. That is rubbish. But it can adversely affect women's sexual confidence and attitudes, particularly when every problem you have is blamed on your hormones.

In fact, menopause and the years beyond should be seen as a time for greater sexual enjoyment. Children are no longer as much of a tie and you don't have to worry about contraception. Some women have an increased sexual drive at this time, because the level of testosterone, the male hormone all women have in their bodies, becomes proportionately higher. The famous anthropologist Margaret Mead called this "post-menopausal zest." Testosterone is linked to motivation and assertiveness as well as sex drive, which may explain why, in traditional cultures, older women are regarded as counselors, leaders and lawmakers. Post-menopausal women can have up to 20 times the amount of testosterone as pre-menopausal women. How's that for the "hormonal deficit" such women are supposed to suffer from?

Both partners may need to make adjustments at menopause. Communication and honesty are the key and can prevent misunderstandings and resentment from building up between you. By communicating honestly about what you like and don't like, changing positions if your favorite one has become uncomfortable and taking the steps recommended to counteract any physical changes, sex should continue to be thoroughly enjoyable. It may take longer, it may be less frequent, and intercourse may not necessarily be the main focus. But although you may have sex less often than you did in your 20s, it can be a deeper, more satisfying experience.

CONTRACEPTION

As a rule of thumb you should wait for two complete period-free years before abandoning contraception if your menopause started before the age of 50. If you were over 50 when it started, a year without periods is considered safe.

VAGINAL DRYNESS

Besides Kegel exercises (see page 195) and vitamin E supplementation (see page 146), lubricants can be helpful. One good one is a pure and natural water-soluble lubricant called Sylk (a product of New Zealand, available online if you can't find it in your local stores).]It does not contain any hormones, drugs or animal products and it is greaseless, non-sticky, stainless and safe to use with condoms.

SEXUAL SATISFACTION

There is no reason why sex should not be as satisfying now as at any other time of your life, and several good reasons why it should be better. Women always take longer to become aroused than men and when you are young the difference can be quite striking. A man in his 20s can achieve orgasm in two to five minutes whereas his partner may take 20 minutes. As a man gets older, he needs longer to reach an orgasm so the timing, in theory, becomes more compatible. The truth is that the aging process has an effect on both men and women, and the so-called "male menopause" may create more problems for your partner than your menopause does for you. Women may worry about their looks but many middle-aged men become very concerned about their sexual performance.

The biggest sexual problem for many women has nothing to do with hormones, vaginal dryness or anything else that can be explained medically. It is boredom. A patient once said to me that HRT was wonderful. Not Hormone Replacement Therapy, she said, but Husband Replacement Therapy. Many women have stayed in a relationship for the sake of their children. Other couples are happy enough but find that passion and excitement has just fizzled out. Once the children grow up and leave home, a couple may find they just don't have much in common any more. This is one reason why women feel they have reached an important turning-point in their lives. Even if they are happy in a relationship, they are conscious of the fact that they have put their children and partners first for as far back as they can remember.

CHAPTER 13

Health Tests at Menopause

There are a number of tests well worth having at menopause because they can assess the state of your health at this crucial time of your life. They can let you know which vitamins you lack and what mineral deficiencies (or surpluses) you may have, and can look at the state of your bones and tell you how well your digestive system is functioning. They can also help you to work out what you might need in the way of food supplements to bring your body back into balance, maintain good health, and help to prevent future problems.

Your health depends on a whole range of factors. Some of these are obvious – diet, lifestyle, stress, age, exercise, addictions (smoking, alcohol, coffee and even tea), environment, constitution and inherited strengths and weaknesses – but others, such as job satisfaction, leisure time, relationships and a sense of purpose and direction, are just as significant. Some of these areas you can control; others you cannot. What many of these tests do is pinpoint the areas where you are not in control and give you an idea of how to redress the balance.

Nowadays, more and more of these tests are performed in your own home. Some, such as the tests for menopausal hormones, diabetes, cholesterol and anemia, give you an instant answer, while with others, a sample is taken at home and sent off to a lab where the results are interpreted by a qualified practitioner. In each case, they give you the knowledge you need to improve your health.

> To obtain the tests mentioned in this chapter, contact www.natural healthpractice.com. The website also contains extensive information on the tests, herbs and supplements recommended throughout the book.

Health tests explained
1 Bones

Many women are concerned about osteoporosis at the time of menopause, and rightly so. Fear of osteoporosis is one of the main reasons why many women choose HRT, but there is no need to feel pressured into taking it. There is now a safe way to find out the condition of your bones.

OSTEOPOROSIS RISK EVALUATION (BONE TURNOVER TEST)

This non-invasive urine test reveals the condition of your bones and assesses your risk of osteoporosis. It gives a dynamic picture of bone turnover by measuring markers in the urine that are excreted as the bone breaks down. If you are losing more bone than you should, you can seek advice on how to slow down the rate of loss and get the most appropriate treatment (see page 89). On the other hand, if your bone health is good, you are in the wonderful position of being able to prevent osteoporosis naturally through diet, supplements and exercise, and by monitoring your bones to make sure they stay healthy.

2 Digestion

Efficient digestion is always important but it is vital during and after menopause because it can help to prevent osteoporosis. Unfortunately, production of

---

How healthy is your digestive system?

- Do you often feel bloated?
- Do you have a full feeling in your stomach, especially after eating?
- Do you often have gas?
- Do you have irritable bowel symptoms, nervous stomach or loose stools?
- Do you avoid certain foods because they make you feel uncomfortable?
- Are you allergic to any foods?
- Have you had any of the following: asthma, allergies, high blood pressure, heart disease, stroke, arthritis, an autoimmune disease (such as rheumatoid arthritis) or yeast infection (like thrush)?
- Have you ever taken an antibiotic for more than one month at a time or have you taken them more than four times in your life?
- Have you ever taken the Pill, HRT or steroids (cortisone, prednisolone etc.) for long periods of time?
- Do you have abdominal cramps or pain?
- Do you get heartburn or indigestion, or belch after meals?
- Have you ever had food poisoning and your bowels have not been "right" since?

If you answered yes to at least two of the questions then your digestive system may be compromised.

stomach acid (hydrochloric acid) decreases with age and this can interfere with the absorption of calcium, which is essential for maintaining strong bones. Other nutrients can be affected too, and if you do not digest and absorb food correctly, you will not benefit from them, no matter how well you eat or what supplements you take. That is why it is important to test for allergies, vitamin and mineral deficiencies, and toxins if you suffer from indigestion.

COMPREHENSIVE DIGESTIVE STOOL ANALYSIS

If you have any of the risk factors for osteoporosis listed on page 83–87, or you have been warned that your bone density is low, and/or you have symptoms of digestive problems, such as bloating, flatulence, irritable bowel syndrome or food allergies, this test could be very helpful. The digestive analysis is performed on a stool sample and includes a group of 25 tests which can evaluate:

- how efficiently you are digesting food molecules (proteins, fats and starches) and absorbing nutrients
- hidden yeast (candida) and bacterial infections
- levels of good bacteria in the digestive tract (intestinal flora balance)
- intestinal immune function
- dietary fiber intake
- the presence of parasites.

FOOD ALLERGY TEST

There are two types of food allergies. Type A (classic allergy) is diagnosed when the reaction takes place immediately after contact with an allergen. Peanuts are a well-known example but others include shellfish and strawberries. In extreme cases, Type A allergy can be fatal, so the only course is to avoid the allergen completely. But there is another form of allergy that is milder, and although it can cause troublesome symptoms, these can be overcome. This Type B delayed allergy (also called food intolerance) causes a reaction one hour to four days after contact with the allergen. Common Type-B allergens include dairy products, eggs, wheat and sugar, which can cause symptoms such as weight gain, bloating, water retention, fatigue, aching joints and headaches.

When food is not digested properly (see Leaky gut test, below) food particles can seep into the bloodstream. Instead of seeing these particles as food, your body views them as toxins and the immune system reacts against them. This is often caused by sheer overload – in other words, eating too much of the same foods too often. Wheat is often a culprit because you may have toast for breakfast, sandwich for lunch, pasta at the evening meal and cookies in between.

To pinpoint what is causing the problem, you can have a blood test that analyzes reactions to different foods and additives. Once you know which foods are causing a reaction, you can avoid them for a short period of time. This gives your body the chance to strengthen and correct any digestive problems so that eventually you can resume eating the foods that used to trigger your allergy (as long as you do so in moderation).

LEAKY GUT TEST

Tracking down the foods to which you are sensitive is only part of the problem, because allergies and food intolerances are often a symptom of underlying illness. The question is, why has the sensitivity developed? And second, what happens when you re-introduce the offending foods? The root cause is the state of the gut and its capacity to process food properly. It is important to investigate this, because if your intestines are not functioning as they should, you may not absorb nutrients efficiently and may become deficient in vital vitamins and minerals.

If your digestive system is working well, the food you eat is broken down thoroughly, passed into the bloodstream, and dealt with successfully by the body's lymphatic system, which helps to remove waste. If this doesn't happen, the body treats normal food as a toxin, and the immune system reacts against it, creating a food allergy. At the same time, this undigested food sits around, fermenting and putrefying. Large spaces can develop between the cells in the gut wall and food molecules can then pass into the bloodstream. This is called leaky gut, or "intestinal permeability," and can result in the overgrowth of candida, or yeast. Banning the offending foods from your diet will help to alleviate the symptoms and make you feel better. But then the whole environment of the gut needs to be healed, to re-establish a healthy level of intestinal bacteria so that you can prevent the symptoms from recurring.

This condition has only recently been widely recognized, so testing for it is relatively new. There is, however, a very simple and effective non-invasive urine test that can be done in your own home. Two urine samples are required. The first is a pre-test sample and the second is taken six hours after drinking a special liquid containing two marker molecules. The samples are sent back to the laboratory and when they are analyzed, the marker molecules are counted. This gives a strong indication as to how "leaky" or permeable your gut is. If the test (which can be arranged by mail) shows that you have a leaky gut, you will be given recommendations and supplement suggestions for healing your digestive system.

3 Hormones

There are two different types of hormone test that are useful around the time of menopause. The first gives a guide to your sex hormones and the second helps to monitor stress levels.

MENOPAUSAL HORMONE TEST

One of the easiest ways to establish whether menopause is starting is to measure the level of the hormone that triggers ovulation. This can show whether symptoms such as erratic or heavy periods and flashes or sweats are the result of menopause or of something else that may need further investigation. A simple urine test performed at home can determine whether you are menopausal. This assesses levels of follicle-stimulating hormone (FSH), which tends to rise dramatically as you approach menopause.

STRESS TEST

This measures the secretion of hormones by the adrenal glands by analyzing four saliva samples taken at home over the course of a day, which are sent to the lab for analysis. In the normal course of events, levels of stress hormones are highest in the morning, giving you the energy you need to face the day, and lowest at night when you want to wind down, ready for bed.

Unfortunately many people are in a constant state of stress, which disrupts the rhythm. This can affect the body in many ways. It can cause lack of energy and you may notice that you find it difficult to get up in the morning. It can increase the risk of osteoporosis, because consistently high levels of the stress hormone cortisol prevent the proper build-up of bone. Your immune system and thyroid function may be compromised, as may your reproductive system, which is especially susceptible to stress, so your periods may stop or become irregular. This effect can last beyond menopause. If they are overtaxed, the adrenals will be unable to produce the estrogen they are designed to supply when your ovaries cease production.

If the test (which again can be arranged by mail) shows that your adrenal glands are overworking, you will be given recommendations and supplement suggestions to help you nourish them and get them working appropriately.

4 Nutrition

Modern life is incredibly busy and there is little time to be choosy about what you eat. Even if your diet is well balanced you may be malnourished, because your health also depends on how well you are able to absorb and digest the nutrients you eat. Unless your digestion works smoothly, you may be deficient in the vitamins and minerals you need to keep your body healthy, and that can cause further problems. Lack of energy, insomnia, headaches, depression, mood swings, anxiety and many other symptoms can be traced directly to deficiencies of specific vitamins and minerals.

Vitamins and minerals work in balance with one another. For this reason, it is vital that you take the right ones in the right amounts, in the right combinations and at the right times. You will notice that each supplement program in this book recommends taking a combined multivitamin and mineral supplement. This is because you need a good foundation, containing all the key nutrients. All nutrients work in harmony and if you take one on its own (such as zinc, for example), you can disturb the balance.

To find out exactly what you need, it is worth taking a test to evaluate your nutritional status.

HAIR ANALYSIS

There are many ways of testing nutritional status – for example, by using a sample of blood or sweat. But one of the most cost-effective and convenient methods involves analyzing your hair, which gives a printout of your mineral and nutritional history.[1] Because your hair contains some of the fastest-growing cells in your body, they "lock in" information about your exposure to certain nutrients as they grow. In this way, your hair forms a permanent record of your exposure to both beneficial and toxic elements.

Hair analysis has great potential for diagnosing disease, and it is possible that it will eventually be used to screen for diabetes and breast cancer. In Australia, Professor Veronica James of the University of New South Wales is attempting to detect these problems by analyzing hair with a technique called X-ray diffraction.[2] As X-rays are fired through the hair, they form a pattern on photographic film that can reveal significant changes. Sugar, for instance, can be found clinging to the hair strands of people with diabetes.

Hair samples can also be used to test for cocaine, amphetamines and cannabis. This is helpful in forensic medicine and pathology and can determine whether someone was under the influence of drugs at the time of an accident. Hair also plays an important part in many medical studies that assess exposure to toxic metals such as mercury, aluminum and cadmium.[3]

Hair analysis is most commonly used in measuring levels of minerals in the body, such as calcium, magnesium, zinc, selenium, copper, manganese and chromium. It has many advantages over other forms of testing. Levels of trace elements such as selenium can be higher in hair, making them easier to detect, and because hair doesn't need specialized sampling equipment or storage, it is convenient for people who do not live near a qualified health practitioner. More importantly, other ways of testing (using blood or urine, for example) may be less reliable because the results are influenced by what is going on in your body at the time. What you have had to eat is one factor, and indulging in a high-fat meal before a cholesterol test will skew the results.

Information may also be misleading when the body attempts to restore balance by topping up the level of nutrients in the blood. If your blood calcium levels fall, for instance, your body will steal calcium from your bones to keep them constant. A blood test may suggest that your calcium levels are fine but a hair test could give quite different results because your hair records what has happened over time rather than what is happening right now. A high level of calcium in your hair could indicate that although there is adequate calcium in the blood, this is because it is being leached from your bones. This information is particularly useful around the time of menopause, when maintaining bone density is crucial. If this leaching effect is seen in a hair test, recommendations can be given to prevent it and to strengthen your bones. Research has shown that abnormal levels of both calcium and phosphorus in hair samples can point to disturbances in bone metabolism,[4] which means that hair analysis can help to identify the cause as well as the presence of health problems.

The results of the test are set out in the form of a graph, so you can see how far your mineral levels differ from the norm. This makes it easy to detect a deficiency of a particular mineral – zinc or selenium, say. Look out for higher-than-average levels too, especially of copper, which can be caused by the Pill, contraceptive coil, HRT and fertility drugs. Excess copper is a concern because it is often associated with zinc deficiency, and zinc is important for the health of the reproductive system.

Apart from detecting imbalances in minerals, hair analysis can also detect high levels of toxic metals such as mercury, cadmium and aluminum. In this case, you should first try to work out the source of contamination and avoid it if possible. You will also need to take specific nutrients, such as antioxidants, to eliminate the toxins from your body.

Of course, there are some drawbacks to hair analysis. Like any testing medium, it has its limitations. Certain minerals (iron, for instance) are best tested by a blood sample. It is important that your hair is not contaminated by tints, highlights or perms for four to six weeks before doing the test.

Swimming can also confuse the analysis. Swimmers' hair may show unusually high levels of copper because the pools are treated with algaecides that alter levels of this mineral.

To address these problems, hair analysis is usually accompanied by a comprehensive questionnaire that asks about your eating habits, lifestyle, symptoms, health problems and risk factors. Each vitamin and mineral has certain deficiency symptoms so a lack of vitamin C, for example, can give you frequent infections, easy bruising, bleeding gums, and slow wound healing. You will be sent a detailed report documenting the 12 vitamins (A, D, E, C, B_1, B_2, B_3, B_5, B_6, B_{12}, folic acid and biotin), seven minerals (calcium, magnesium, zinc, manganese, copper, chromium and selenium) and essential fatty acids you need to take, and specifying the quantities required for optimum health. You are usually advised to repeat the hair test after following the recommendations for three to four months. Once your levels are back to normal, it is important to keep to a maintenance program and to continue to eat well.

For further information on any of these tests, please contact me or see my website (see page 236).

The Future

Since 1997, my conviction that our first choice should always be the natural approach has been strengthened. Menopause is a natural event and HRT should remain the last resort.

In today's world, our bodies are bombarded by many different substances. Our food can contain a cocktail of chemicals in the form of additives and preservatives, and may well be genetically modified or irradiated. On top of this, there are all the toxins and pollutants that we are exposed to, which include xenoestrogens. We are asking a lot for our bodies by expecting them to deal with all this. To try to keep healthy, we should make things as easy for ourselves as possible. Adding in more substances in the form of hormones only serves to increase our body's workload.

It is important that we make informed decisions about our health. We are all individuals with different medical histories and genetic legacies. These factors have to be taken into account in order to meet our own particular circumstances.

Ask your health care professional all the questions you want. Remember that it is your body and if you are offered treatment, you need to know of any possible side effects. So eat well, keep fit and stay healthy.

Suggested further reading

Books on menopause
Coney, Sandra *The Menopause Industry* (Hunter House, 1994)
Love, Susan *Dr. Susan Love's Breast Book* (Perseus Publishing, 2000)
Northrup, Christiane *The Wisdom of Menopause* (Doubleday, 2003)

Food and cooking
Glenville, Marilyn *Eat Your Way Through the Menopause* (Kyle Cathie, 2002)

General health
Cadbury, Deborah *Feminization of Nature* (St. Martin's Press, 1999)
Carson, Rachel *Silent Spring* (Mariner Books, 2002)
Colborn, Theo, Dianne Dumanoski and John Peterson *Our Stolen Future* (Plume, 1997)
Glenville, Marilyn *Natural Alternatives to Dieting* (Kyle Cathie, 1999)
————————, *The Nutritional Health Handbook for Women* (Piatkus, 2001)

Useful addresses

Acupuncture
American Academy of Medical
Acupuncture Physicians
4929 Wilshire Boulevard, Suite 428
Los Angeles, CA 90010-3817
Tel: 800-521-2262
www.medicalacupuncture.org

Homeopathy
National Center for Homeopathy
801 North Fairfax Street, Suite 306
Alexandria, VA 22314
Tel: 703-548-7790
www.homeopathic.org

Medical Herbalism
Herb Research Foundation
1007 Pearl Street, Suite 200
Boulder, CO 80302
Tel: 303-449-2265
www.herbs.org

Nutrition
American Dietetic Association
120 South Riverside Plaza, Suite 2000
Chicago, IL 60606
Tel: 800-877-1600
www.eatright.org

Osteopathy
American Academy of Osteopathy (AAO)
3500 DePauw Boulevard, Suite 1080
Indianapolis, IN 46268-1136
Tel: 317-879-1881
www.academyofosteopathy.org

Osteoporosis
National Osteoporosis Foundation
1232 22nd Street Northwest
Washington, D.C. 20037
Tel: 202-223-2226
www.nof.org

Premature menopause
The Daisy Network
PO BOX 392
High Wycombe, Bucks
England HP15 7SH

Premature Ovarian Failure
Support Group
P.O. Box 23643
Alexandria, VA 22304
Tel: 703-913-4787
www.pofsupport.org

Yoga
Yoga Journal
2054 University Avenue
Berkeley, CA 94704
www. yogajournal.com

References

Introduction
1. Cooper, J. and Marsh, J. (1999), *Maturitas*, 15, 151-8 and "Achieving long-term compliance of menopausal HRT" (North American Menopause Society Consensus Opinion, 1998) *Menopause*, 5, 69-76

Chapter 1
1. Goldfarb, H.A. (1997), *The No-Hysterectomy Option*, John Wiley & Sons

Chapter 3
1. Finn, C.A. (2002), "Why do women have a menopause?," *Journal of the British Menopause Society*, 8, 1, 10–14
2. Diamond, J. (1996), "Why Women Change," *Discover*, 131-7
3. Hoover, R. *et al* (1976), *New England Journal of Medicine*, 295, 401-5
4. Ziel, H. and Finkle, H. (1975), *New England Journal of Medicine*, 293, 1167-70
5. Crook, D. (1999), "Will the route of administration influence the potential cardiovascular benefits of postmenopausal HRT?," *Journal of the British Menopause Society*, 5, 35-9
6. Okon, M.A. (1997), "Period-free hormone replacement therapy," *Journal of the British Menopause Society*, 3,1, 11-14
7. McCullough, W. and Gangar, K. (1998), "Problems with HRT," *The Diplomate – The Journal of the Diplomates of the Royal College of Obstetricians and Gynaecologists*, 5, 1, 33–6
8. Gangar, K.F. *et al* (1990), "Prolonged endometrial stimulation associated with oestradiol implants," *British Medical Journal*, 300, 436-8
9. McCullough, W. and Gangar, K. (1998), "Problems with HRT Minisymposium: oestradiol implants, supraphysiological oestradiol levels, withdrawal and tachyphylaxis," *The Diplomate*, 5, 1, 33-6
10. Willhite, S.L. *et al* (1998), Raloxifene provides an alternatives for osteoporosis prevent. *Ann Pharmacother*, 32, 834-7
11. Ettinger, B. *et al* (1999), "Reduction of vertebral fracture risk in postmenopausal women with osteoporosis treated with Raloxifene: results from a 3 year randomised clinical trial. Multiple Outcomes of Raloxifene Evaluation (MORE) Investigators," *Journal of the American Medical Association*, 282, 637-45
12. Hall, J.M. and McDonnell, D.P. (1999), "The oestrogen receptor beta-isoform (ERbeta) of the human oestrogen receptor modulates ERalpha transcriptional activity and is a key regulator of the cellular response to oestrogens and antioestrogens," *Endocrinology*, 140, 12, 5566-78
13. Brezinski (1999), "Phytoestrogens, the "natural' SERMS?," *European Journal of Obstetrics and Gynaecology*, 85, 47-51.
14. Hoover, R. *et al*, *New England Journal of Medicine*, 1976, 295: 401-5.
15. Beral, V. (1997), "Breast cancer and HRT: collaborative reanalysis of data from 51 epidemiological studies of 52,705 women with breast cancer and 108,411 without breast cancer," *The Lancet*, 350, 1047-59
16. Schairer, C. (2000), "Menopausal oestrogen and oestrogen-progestogen replacement therapy and breast cancer risk," *Journal of the American Medical Association*, 283, 4, 485-91
17. Writing Group for the Women's Health Initiative Investigators (2002), "Risks and benefits of oestrogen plus progestin in healthy postmenopausal women: principal results from the Women's Health Initiative randomised controlled trial," *Journal of the American Medical Association*, 288, 321-33
18. Ozdemir, A. *et al* (1999), "Mammographic and ultrasonographic study of changes in the breast related to HRT," *International Journal of Gynaecology and Obstetrics*, 67, 23-32
19. Slanetz, P.J. (2002), "Hormone replacement therapy and breast tissue density on mammography," *Menopause: The Journal of the North American Menopause Society*, 9, 2, 82-3
20. Christodoulakos, G.E. (2002), "Mammographic changes associated with Raloxifene and Tibolone therapy in postmenopausal women: a prospective study," *Menopause: The Journal of the North American Menopause Society*, 9, 2, 110-16
21. Smith et al (1975), *New England Journal of Medicine*, 293, 1164-7
22. Grady, D. et al (1995), "Hormone replacement therapy and endometrial cancer risk: a meta-analysis," *Obstetrics and Gynaecology*, 85, 2, 304-13
23. Miller, J. et al (2002), "Postmenopausal oestrogen replacement and risk for venous

thromboembolism: a systematic review and meta-analysis for the US Preventive Services Task Force," *Annals of Internal Medicine*, 136, 680-90

24. Grady, D. *et al* (2000), "Postmenopausal hormone therapy increases risk for venous thromboembolic disease: the Heart and Oestrogen/progestin Replacement Study," *Annals of International Medicine*, 132, 689-96

25. Writing Group for the Women's Health Initiative Investigators (2002), "Risks and benefits of oestrogen plus progestin in healthy postmenopausal women: principal results from the Women's Health Initiative randomised controlled trial," *Journal of the American Medical Association*, 288, 321-33

26. Grodstein et al (1996), "Prospective study of exogenous hormones and risk of pulmonary embolism in women," *The Lancet*, 348, 983-7

27. Antiplatelet Trialists' Collaboration (1994), "Collaborative overview of randomised trials of antiplatelet therapy III. Reduction in venous thrombosis and pulmonary embolism by antiplatelet prophylaxis against surgical and medical patients," *British Medical Journal*, 308, 235-46

28. Hulley *et al* (1998), "Randomised trial of oestrogen plus progestin for secondary prevention of coronary heart disease in postmenopausal women," *Journal of the American Medical Association*, 280, 605-13

29. Bosetti, C. *et al* (2001), "Relationship between postmenopausal hormone replacement therapy and ovarian cancer," Journal of the American Medical Association, 285, 24, 3089

30. Editorial, *The Lancet* (2002), 359, 9313

31. Dawson-Hughes, B. *et al* (1997), "Effect of calcium and vitamin D supplementation on bone density in men and women 65 years of age or older," *New England Journal of Medicine*, 337, 670-6

32. Mosekilde, L. et al (2000), Hormonal replacement therapy reduces forearm fracture incidence in recent postmenopausal women: results of the Danish Osteoporosis Prevention Study," *Maturitas*, 36, 181-93

33. Writing Group for the Women's Health Initiative Investigators (2002), "Risks and benefits of oestrogen plus progestin in healthy postmenopausal women: principal results from the Women's Health Initiative randomised controlled trial," *Journal of the American Medical Association*, 288, 321-33

34. Michaelsson, K. *et al* (1998), "Hormone replacement therapy and the risk of hip fracture: Population-based case-control study," *British Medical Journal*, 316, 1858-63

35. Hulley *et al* (1998), "Randomised trial of oestrogen plus progestin for secondary prevention of coronary heart disease in postmenopausal women," *Journal of the American Medical Association*, 280, 605-613 and The Writing Group for the PEPI (1996) "Effects of hormone therapy on bone mineral density: results from the postmenopausal oestrogen/progestin interventions (PEPI) trial," *Journal of the American Medical Association*, 276, 1389-96

36. Grady, D. and Cummings, S.R. (2001), "Postmenopausal hormone therapy for prevention of fractures: how good is the evidence?," *Journal of the American Medical Association*, 285, 22, 2909-10

37. Mulnard *et al*, Journal of the American Medical Association, 2000, 283, 1007

38. *Journal of the American Medical Association*, 2002, 287, 591-7

39. Grady, D. *et al* (2001), "Postmenopausal hormones and incontinence: the Heart and Estrogen/Progestin Replacement Study," *Obstetrics and Gynaecology*, 97, 116-20

40. Writing Group for the Women's Health Initiative Investigators (2002), "Risks and benefits of oestrogen plus progestin in healthy postmenopausal women: principal results from the Women's Health Initiative randomised controlled trial," *Journal of the American Medical Association*, 288, 321-33

41. Casper, R.F. *et al* (1979), "Menopausal flushes: A neuroendocrine link with pulsatile luteinising hormone secretion," *Science*, 205, 823-5

Chapter 4

1. Wren, B.G. (2001), Transdermal progesterone or synthetic progestogens, *Journal of the British Menopause Society*, 7, 3, 115-118

2. Kim, S. *et al* (1996), "Antiproliferative effects of low-dose micronized progesterone, *Fertility and Sterility*, 65, 2, 323-31

3. Grimes, D. (1992), *Fertility and Sterility*, 57, 3, 492-3

4. Horwitz, K.B. *et al* (1995), "Surprises with antiprogestins: Novel mechanisms of progesterone receptor action," *Ciba Foundation Symposium*, 191: 235-49; (discussion) 250-3

5. *International Journal of Cancer* (2001), 92, 469–73
6. Hyder, S.M. *et al* (2001), "Pharmacological and endogenous prostegins induce vascular endothelial growth factor expression in human breast cells," *International Journal of Cancer*, 92, 4, 469–73

Chapter 5

1. Upmalis, D. *et al* (2000), "Vasomotor symptom relief by soy isoflavone extract tablets in postmenopausal women: a multicentre, double-blind, randomised, placebo-controlled study," *Menopause*, 7, 4, 2236–42
2. Albertazzi, P. *et al* (1998), "The effect of dietary soy supplementation on hot flushes," *Obstetrics and Gynaecology*, 91, 1
3. *Journal of Nutrition* (1995), 125, 437–45
4. Kessel, B. (1996), "Alternatives to oestrogen for menopausal women," *Proceedings of the Society for Experimental Biology and Medicine*, 217, 38–44
5. Boulet, M. (1994), "Climacteric and menopause in seven south-east Asian countries," *Maturitas*, 19, 157–76
6. Coleman, M.P. *et al* (1993), "Trends in cancer incidence and mortality, Lyon, France," *IARC Publications*, no. 121
7. de Kleijn, M.J. *et al* (2001), "Intake of dietary phytoestrogens is low in postmenopausal women in the United States: the Framingham study," *Journal of Nutrition*, 131, 6, 1826–32
8. Phillimore, Jane, "Soya Bean Crisis," *The Observer Magazine*, 27 August 2000
9. Lappe, M.A. *et al* (1999), "Alterations in clinically important phytoestrogens in genetically modified, herbicide-tolerant soybeans," *Journal of Medicinal Food*, 1, 4
10. Aldecreutz, H. (1988), "Lignans and phytoestrogens: possible preventive role in cancer," in P. Rozen, ed, *Frontiers of Gastrointestinal Research*, vol. 14, 165–76, Karger, Basel, Switzerland

Chapter 6

1. Budd, M. (1995), *Low Blood Sugar*, Thorsons
2. Ringsdorf, W. et al (1976), "Sucrose, neutrophil phagocytosis and resistance to disease," *Dental Survey*, 52, 46–8
3. Blundell, J.E. and Hill, A.J. (1986), "Paradoxical effects of an intense sweetener (aspartame) on appetite," *The Lancet*, 1, 1092–3
4. Wurtman, R.J. (1983), "Neurochemical changes following high dose aspartame with dietary carbohydrates," *New England Journal of Medicine*, 429–30
5. Stegink, L.D. *et al* (1989), "Effect of repeated ingestion of aspartame-sweetened beverage on plasma amino acid, blood methanol and blood formate concentrations," *Metabolism*, 38, 4, 357–63
6. Lipton, S.A. and Rosenberg, P.A. (1994), "Excitatory amino acids as a final common pathway for neurologic disorders," *New England Journal of Medicine*, 300, 9, 613–22
7. *The Lancet*, 21 May 1994
8. Lappe, M.A. et al (1999), "Alterations in clinically important phytoestrogens in genetically modified, herbicide-tolerant soybeans," *Journal of Medicinal Food*, 1, 4

Chapter 7

1. Jonsson, B. *et al* (1999), "Effect and offset of treatments for hip fracture on health outcomes," *Osteoporosis International*, 10, 193–9
2. Gail, A. *et al* (2000), "How many women lose bone mineral density while taking hormone replacement therapy? Results from the Postmenopausal Estrogen/Progestin Interventions Trial," *Archives of Internal Medicine*, 160, 3065–71
3. Kanis, J. (2000), *Journal of the British Menopause Society*, Supplement 2, vol 5, 17–19
4. Lips, P. (1997), "Epidemiology and predictors of fractures associated with osteoporosis," *American Journal of Medicine*, 103, 3S–8S
5. Lees, B. *et al* (1993), "Differences in proximal femur bone density over two centuries," *The Lancet*, 341, 8846, 673–5
6. World Health Organization, "Assessment of fracture risk and its application to screening for post-menopausal osteoporosis," Geneva: WHO, 1994 (Technical report series 843)
7. Carmichael, K.A. and Carmichae, D.H. (1995), "Bone metabolism and osteopenia in eating disorders," *Medicine*, 74, 254–67
8. Kiriike, N. *et al* (1992), "Reduced bone density and major hormones regulating calcium

metabolism in anorexia nervosa" *Acta Psychiatrica Scandinavica*, 86, 358–65

9. Kin *et al* (1991), *Calcification Tissue International*, 49, 101–6

10. Law, M.R. and Hackshaw, A.K. (1997), "A meta-analysis of cigarette smoking, bone mineral density and risk of hip fracture: recognition of a major effect," *British Medical Journal*, 315, 841–6

11. Jick *et al* (1977), "Relation between smoking and age of natural menopause," *The Lancet*, 1, 1354–5

12. Francis, R. (1998), "Management of corticosteroid-induced osteoporosis," *Journal of the British Menopause Society*, 4,2, 52–6

13. *New England Journal of Medicine* (2001), 345, 941–7

14. Bauer, D.C. *et al* (1992), "Hyperthyroidism increases the risk of osteoporotic hip fractures. A prospective study," *Journal of Bone and Mineral Research*, 7, S121

15. Xiaoge, D. *et al* (2000), "Bone mineral density differences at the femoral neck and Ward's triangle: a comparison study on the reference data between Chinese and Caucasian women," *Calcification Tissue International*, 67, 195–8

16. Wilkins, T.J. (1999), "Changing perceptions in osteoporosis," *British Medical Journal*, 318, 862–5

17. Kanis, J.A. and Gluer, C.C. (2000), "An update on the diagnosis and assessment of osteoporosis with densitometry," Committee of Scientific Advisors, International Osteoporosis Foundation. *Osteoporosis International*, 11, 192–202.

18. Eastell, R. and Bainbridge, P. (2001), "Bone turnover markers for monitoring antiresorptive therapy," *Osteoporosis Review*, 9, 1, 1–5

19. Melton, L.J. III *et al* (1997), "Relationship of bone turnover to bone density and fracture," *Journal of Bone Mineral Research*, 12, 7, 1083–91

20. Hans, D. *et al* (1996), "Ultrasonographic heel measurements to predict hip fracture in elderly women: the EPIDOS study," *The Lancet*, 348, 511–14

21. Position statement on the use of quantitative ultrasound in the management of osteoporosis, National Osteoporosis Society, December, 2001

22. Faulkner, K.G. (2000), "Bone matters: are density increases necessary to reduce fracture risk?," *Journal of Bone Mineral Research*, 15, 183–7 and Wilkins, T.J. (1999), "Changing perceptions in osteoporosis," British Medical Journal, 318, 862–5

23. Lin, J.H. (1996), "Biphosphonates: a review of their pharmacokinetic properties," *Bone*, 18, 75–85

24. Hosking, D. et al (1998), "Prevention of bone loss with alendronate in postmenopausal under 60 years of age," *New England Journal of Medicine*, 338, 485–92

25. Harris, S.T. *et al* (1999), "Effects of risedronate treatment on vertebral and nonvertebral fractures in women with postmenopausal osteoporosis: a randomised controlled trial," Vertebral Efficacy with Risedronate Therapy (VERT) Study Group, *Journal of the American Medical Association*, 282, 1344–52

26. Kurttio, P. *et al* (1999), "Exposure to natural fluoride in well water and hip fracture: a cohort analysis in Finland" *American Journal of Epidemiology*, 150, 817–24

27. Goldsmith *et al* (1976), "Effects of phosphorus supplementation on serum parathyroid hormone and bone morphology in osteoporosis," *Journal of Clinical Endocrinology and Metabolism*, 523–32

28. Kerstetter, J.E. et al (1999), "Changes in bone turnover in young women consuming different levels of dietary protein," *Journal of Clinical Endocrinology and Metabolism*, 84, 1052–5

29. Feskanich *et al* (1996), "Protein Consumption and Bone Fractures in Women," *American Journal of Epidemiology*, 143, 5, 472–9

30. Sanchez, V. *et al* (1978), "Bone mineral mass in elderly vegetarian females," *American Journal of Roentgenol*, 131, 542

31. Ellis, F. *et al* (1972), "Incidence of osteoporosis in vegetarians and omnivores," *American Journal of Clinical Nutrition*, 25, 55–8

32. Saffar, J.L. *et al* (1981), "Osteoporotic effect of a high carbohydrate diet in golden hamsters," *Archives of Oral Biology*, 26, 393–7

33. Holbook, T.L. and Barrett-Conner, E. (1993), *British Medical Journal*, 1056–8

34. Hegarty, V. *et al* (2000), "Tea drinking and bone mineral density in older women," *American Journal of Clinical Nutrition*, 71, 1003–7

35. Basu, S. *et al* (2001), "Association between oxidative stress and bone mineral density," *Biochemical and Biophysical Research Communications*, 288, 1, 275–9

36. Felson, D. *et al* (1988), "Alcohol consumption and hip fractures: The Framingham study," *American Journal of Epidemiology*, 128, 1102-10

37. Goulding, A. (1990), "Osteoporosis: why consuming less sodium chloride helps to conserve bone," *New Zealand Medical Journal*, 102, 12-122

38. Tucker, K.L. *et al* (1999), "Potassium, Magnesium and Fruit and Vegetable Intakes are associated with greater bone mineral density in elderly men and women," *American Journal of Clinical Nutrition*, 69, 4, 727-36

39. Cooper et al (1992), Osteoporosis, 285-9, and "High soya consumption is associated with increased bone mass," *Obstetrics and Gynaecology* (2001), 97, 1, 109-15

40. Potter, S.M. *et al* (1998), "Soy protein and isoflavones: their effects on blood lipids and bone density in postmenopausal women," *American Journal of Clinical Nutrition*, 68(S), 1375S-1379S

41. Rico, H. *et al* (2000), "Effect of silicon supplement on osteopenia induced by ovariectomy in rats," *Calcification Tissue International*, 66, 53-5

42. Damien, D. (2001) "Vitamin D – Time for Reassessment," *Journal of Nutritional and Environmental Medicine*, 11, 237-9

43. Dawson-Hughes, B. *et al* (2000), "Effect of withdrawal of calcium and vitamin D supplements on bone mass in elderly men and women," *American Journal of Clinical Nutrition*, 72, 745-50

44. Brattstrom, L. *et al* (1985), "Folic acid responsive postmenopausal homocysteinemia," *Metabolism*, 1073-7

45. Benke, P.J. *et al* (1972), "Osteoporotic bone disease in the pyridoxine-deficient rat," *Biochemical Medicine*, 6, 526-35

46. Kanai, T. *et al* (1997), "Serum vitamin K level and bone mineral density in post-menopausal women," *International Journal of Gynaecology and Obstetrics*, 56, 25-30

47. Current Research in Osteoporosis and Bone Mineral Measurement II, British Institute of Radiology, 1992

48. Sojka, J.E. (1995), "Magnesium supplementation and osteoporosis," Nutrition Reviews, 53, 71-80

49. Creedon, A. *et al* (1999), "The effect of moderately and severely restricted dietary magnesium intakes on bone composition and bone metabolism in the rate," *British Journal of Nutrition*, 82, 63-71

50. Stending-Lindberg, G. *et al* (1993), "Trabecular bone density in a two year controlled trial of personal magnesium in osteoporosis," *Magnesium Research*, 6, 155-63

51. Sakhaee, K. *et al* (1999), "Meta-analysis of calcium bioavailability: a comparison of calcium citrate and calcium carbonate," *American Journal of Therapeutics*, 5, 313-21

52. Carr, C.J. and Shangraw, R.F. (1987), "Nutritional and pharmaceutical aspects of calcium supplementation, *American Pharmacy*, 27, 49-57

53. O'Shea, B. *et al* (2000), "A meta-analysis of calcium supplementation for the prevention of postmenopausal osteoporosis," *Osteoporosis International*, 11, S114

54. Hegsted, D.M. (2001), "Fractures, calcium and the modern diet," *American Journal of Clinical Nutrition*, 74, 5, 571-3

55. Prentice, A. *et al* (1991), "Bone mineral content of British and rural Gambian women aged 18-80+ years," *Bone Mineral*, 12, 3, 201-14

56. Neilsen, F.H. *et al* (1987), "Effect of dietary boron on mineral, oestrogen and testosterone metabolism in postmenopausal women," *FASEB J*, 1, 394-97

57. Penland, J.G. (1998), "The importance of boron nutrition for brain and psychological function," *Biological Trace Element Research,* 66, 299-317

58. Calhoun, N.R. *et al* (1975), "The effects of zinc on ectopic bone formation," *Oral Surgery* 39, 698-706

59. Atik, O.S. (1983), "Zinc and senile osteoporosis," *Journal of the American Geriatric Society*, 31, 790-91

60. Schreiber, M.D. and Rebar, R.W.F. (1999), "Isoflavones and postmenopausal bone health: a viable alternative to oestrogen therapy," *Menopause*, 6, 3, 233-41

61. Alexandersen, P. (2001), "Ipriflavone in the treatment of postmenopausal osteoporosis: a randomised controlled trial. Ipriflavone Multicentre European Fracture Study," *Journal of the American Medical Association*, 285, 1482-8

62. Halpner, A.D. *et al* (2000), "The effect of an ipriflavone-containing supplement on urinary N-linked telopeptide levels in postmenopausal women," *Journal of Women's Health and Gender Based Medicine*, 9, 995-8

63. Kruger, M.C. (1998), "Calcium, gamma-linolenic acid and eicosapentaenoic acid supplementation in senile osteoporosis," *Ageing* (Milano), 10, 385-94

64. Melhus, H. *et al* (1998), "Excessive dietary intake of vitamin A is associated with reduced bone mineral density and increased risk for hip fracture," *Annals of International Medicine*, 129, 770-8

65. Feskanich, D. *et al* (2002), "Vitamin A intake and hip fractures among postmenopausal women," *Journal of the American Medical Association*, 287, 1, 47-54

66. Ibid.

Chapter 8

1. Zhao, G. *et al* (2000), "Menopausal symptoms: experience of Chinese women," *Climacteric*, 3, 2, 135-44

2. Kremer, J. *et al* (1985), "Effects of manipulation of dietary fatty acids on clinical manifestation of rheumatoid arthritis," *The Lancet*, I, 184-7

3. Pujalte, J.M. *et al* (1980), "Double blind clinical evaluation of oral glucosamine sulphate in the basic treatment of osteoarthrosis," *Current Medical Research Opinion*, 7, 2, 110-14

4. Taussig, S.J. and Batkin, S. (1988), "Bromelain, the enzyme complex of pineapple (Ananas comosus) and its clinical application," *Ethnopharmacol*, 1988, 22, 191-203

5. Schellenberg, R. (2001), "Treatment for the pre-menstrual syndrome with agnus fruit extract: prospective, randomised, placebo controlled study," *British Medical Journal*, 322, 134-7

6. Minton, J.P. *et al* (1981), "Clinical and biochemical studies of methylxanthine-related fibrocystic breast disease," *Surgery*, 90, 299-304

7. Petrakis, N.L. and King, E.B. (1981), "Cytological abnormalities in nipple aspirates of breast fluid from women with severe constipation," *The Lancet*, ii, 1, 203-5

8. Boyd, E.M.F. *et al* (1988), "The effect of a low-fat, high complex carbohydrate diet on symptoms of cyclical mastopathy," *The Lancet*, 2, 128-32

9. Wagner, H. (1981) in J.L. Beal and E. Reinhard (eds.), *Natural Products as Medicinal Agents*

10. Halsaka, M. *et al* (1998), "Treatment of cyclical mastodynia using an extract of Vitex agnus-castus: results of a double-blind comparison with placebo," *Ceska Gynekol*, 63, 388-89

11. Linde, E. *et al* (1996), "St John's wort for depression - an overview and meta-analysis of randomised clinical trials," *British Medical Journal*, 313, 253-61

12. Woelk, H. (2000), "Comparison of St John's wort and imipramine for treating depression: randomised controlled trial," *British Medical Journal*, 321, 536-9

13. Johnson, E.J. *et al* (1985), Efficacy of feverfew as prophylactic treatment of migraine, *British Medical Journal*, 291, 569-73

14. Lithgow, D. and Politzer, W. (1977), "Vitamin A in the treatment of Menorrhagia," *South African Medical Journal* 51, 191-3

15. Cohen, J. and Rubin, H. (1960), "Functional Menorrhagia, treatment with bioflavonoids and vitamin C," *Current Therapeutic Research* 2, 11, 539-42

16. Irvin, J.H. *et al* (1996), "The effects of relaxation response training on menopausal symptoms," *Journal of Psychosomatic Obstetrics and Gynaecology*, 17, 202-7

17. Barton, D.L. *et al* (1998), Prospective evaluation of vitamin E for hot flushes in breast cancer survivors," *et al*, 16, 495-500

18. Smith, C. (1964), Non-hormonal control of vaso-motor flushing in menopausal patients, *Chicago Medicine*, 67, 193-5

19. Lieberman, S. (1998), "A review of the effectiveness of Cimicifuga racemosa (black cohosh) for the symptoms of menopause," *Journal of Women's Health*, 75, 5, 525-9

20. Nagata, C. *et al* (2001), "Soy product intake and hot flashes in Japanese women: results from a community-based prospective study," *American Journal of Epidemiology*, 153, 8, 790-3

21. Han, K.K. *et al* (2002), "Benefits of soy isoflavone therapeutic regimen on menopausal symptoms," *Obstetrics and Gynaecology*, 99, 389-94

22. St Germain, A. *et al* (2001), "Isoflavone-rich or isoflavone-poor soy protein does not reduce menopausal symptoms during 24 weeks of treatment," *Menopause*, 8, 17-26

23. Barber, R. *et al* (1999), Randomised placebo-controlled trial of an isoflavone supplement and menopausal symptoms in women, *Climacteric*, 2, 85-92 and Knight, D. *et al* (1999), "The effect of Promensil, an isoflavone extract, on menopausal symptom," *Climacteric*, 2, 79-84

24. Bennetts, H.W. *et al* (1956), "A specific breeding problem of sheep on subterranean clover pastures in Western Australia," *Australian Journal of Agricultural Research*, 22, 131-8

25. File, S.E. *et al* (2001), "Eating soya improves human memory," *Psychopharmacology* (Berl), 157, 4, 430–6
26. Penland, J.G. (1998), "The importance of boron nutrition for brain and psychological function," *Biological Trace Element Research*, 66, 299–317
27. Dellas, A. and Drewe, J. (1995), "Conservative therapy of female genuine stress incontinence with vaginal cones," *European Journal of Obstetrics and Gynaecology and Reproductive Biology*, 62, 213–15
28. Dalais, F.S. *et al* (1998), "Effects of dietary phytoestrogens in postmenopausal women," *Climacteric*, 1, 124–9
29. McLaren, H. (1949), "Vitamin E in the menopause," *British Medical Journal*, 1378–82).

Chapter 9

1. *The Lancet*, 2001, 358, 1389–99
2. Coleman M.P. *et al* (1993), "Trends in Cancer Incidence and Mortality, Lyon, France," *IARC Publication*, 1213. Presented at the European Society for Therapeutic Radiology and Oncology, 1996
4. Schairer, C. (2000), "Menopausal oestrogen and oestrogen–progestogen replacement therapy and cancer," *Journal of the American Medical Association*, 283, 4, 485–91
5. Beral, V. *et al* (2002), Evidence from randomised trials on the longterm effects of HRT, *The Lancet*, 360, 9337, 942
6. Aronson, K.J. (2000), "Breast adipose tissue concentrations of polychlorinated biphenyls and other organochlorines and breast cancer risk," *Cancer Epidemiol Biomarkers Prev*, 9, 1, 55–63
7. Gonazalez, E.R. (1980), "Vitamin E relieves most cystic breast disease; may alter lipids, Hormone," *Journal of the American Medical Association*, 244, 10, 1077–8
8. Miller, A.B. *et al* (1992), "Canadian National Breast Screening Study: 2-breast cancer detection and death rates among women 50 to 59 year," *Canadian Medical Association*, 147, 1477–88
9. Sjonell, G. and Stahle, L. (1999), "Halsokontroller med mammografi minskar inte dodlighet i brostcancer," *Lakartidningen*, 96, 904–13
10. Gotzsche, P.C. and Olsen, O. (2000), "Is screening for breast cancer with mammography justifiable?," *The Lancet*, 355, 129–34
11. Olsen, O. and Gotzsche, P.C. (2001), "Cochrane review on screening for breast cancer with mammography," *The Lancet*, 358, 1340–2
12. Ibid.
13. Colacurci, N. *et al* (2001), "Fewer mammographic density increases seen in women who suspend HRT," *Fertility and Sterility*, 76, 451–5
14. James, V. (1999), "Using hair to screen for breast cancer," *Nature*, 398, 6722, 33–34
15. Cuzick, J. *et al* (1998), "Electropotential measurements as a new diagnostic modality for breast cancer," *The Lancet*, 352, 359
16. Herbert, J. and Rosen, A. (1996), "Nutritional, socioeconomic, and reproductive factors in relation to female breast cancer mortality: findings from a cross-national study," *Cancer Detection and Prevention*, 20, 3, 234–44
17. Boyd, N.F. and McGuire, V. (1991), "The possible role of lipid peroxidation in breast cancer risk," *Free Radical Biology and Medicine*, 10, 3–4, 185–90
18. Winston, R. *et al* (1994), "Regulation of insulin-like growth factors by antioestrogen," *Breast Cancer Research Treatment*, 31, 107–15
19. Kaiser, L. *et al* (1989), "Fish consumption and breast cancer risk," *Nutrition and Cancer*, 12, 61–8
20. Willett, W.C. (1997), "Fat, energy and breast cancer," *Journal of Nutrition*, 127, 5, 921S–923S
21. Chen, C. *et al* (1992), "Antioxidant status and cancer mortality in China," *International Journal of Epidemiology*, 21, 4, 625–35
22. *Journal of Nutrition* (2002), 132, 303–6
23. Lockwood, K. et al (1994), "Apparent partial remission of breast cancer in "high risk" patients supplemented with nutritional antioxidants, essential fatty acids and co-enzyme Q10, *Molecular Aspects of Medicine*, vol 15 (Supplement), s231–s240
24. Aldercreutz *et al* (1992), "Dietary phytoestrogens and cancer: in vitro and in vivo studies," *Journal of Steroid Chemistry and Molecular Biology*, 3–8, 41, 331–7
25. Anderson, J.J.B. *et al* (1999), "Health potential of soy isoflavones for menopausal women,"

Public Health Nutrition, 2, 4, 489–504

26. Barnes, S. (1997), "The chemopreventive properties of soy isoflavonoids in animal models of breast cancer," *Breast Cancer Research and Treatment*, 46, 169–79

27. McMichael, P.D.F. *et al* (1998), "Effects of soy protein supplementation on epithelial proliferation in the histologically normal human breast," *American Journal of Clinical Nutrition*, 68S, S1431–S1436

28. Zava, D. (1998), "Oestrogen and progestogen bioactivity of different foods, spices and herbs," *Proceedings of the Society for Experimental Biology and Medicine*, 217, 369–78

29. Setchell, K.D.R. *et al* (2001), "Bioavailability of pure isoflavones in healthy humans and analysis of commercial soy isoflavone supplements," *American Society for Nutritional Sciences*, 1362S–1375S

30. Amato, P. *et al* (2002), "Oestrogenic activity of herbs commonly used as remedies for menopausal symptoms," *Menopause*, 9, 145–50

31. Nesselhut, T. *et al* (1993), "Examination of the proliferative potential of phytopharmaceuticals with oestrogen-mimicking actions in breast carcinoma," *Archives of Gynaecology and Obstetrics*, 254, 817–18

32. The Endogenous Hormones and Breast Cancer Collaborative Group" (2002), "Endogenous hormones and breast cancer in Postmenopausal women: reanalysis of nine prospective studies," *Journal of the National Cancer Institute*, 94, 8, 606–16

33. Bernstein, L. (1994), *Journal of the National Cancer Institute*, 86, 18

34. Singer, R. and Grismaijer (1995), S. "Dressed to Kill – the link between breast cancer and bras," Avery

35. Schrumpf, F. and Charley, H. (1975), "Texture of broccoli and carrots cooked by microwave energy," *Journal of Food Science*, 40, 1025–9

36. Aronson, K.J. (2000), "Breast adipose tissue concentrations of polychlorinatd biphenyls and other organochlorines and breast cancer risk," *Cancer Epidemiol Biomarkers Prev*, 9, 1, 55–63

37. Verma, S.P. (1997), "Curcumin and genistein, plant natural products, show synergistic inhibitory effects on the growth of human breast cancer MCF-7 cells," *Biophysical Research Communications*, 233, 3, 692–6

Chapter 10

1. Stampfer, M.J. *et al*, *New England Journal of Medicine*, 1985, 313: 1044–9

2. Hulley, S. *et al* (1998), "Randomised trial of oestrogen plus progestogen for secondary prevention of coronary heart disease in postmenopausal women," *Journal American Medical Association*, 280, 6-5-13

3. Mosca, L, *et al* (2001), "Hormone replacement and cardiovascular disease: a statement for healthcare professionals from the American Heart Association," *Circulation*, 104, 499–503

4. Grady, D. *et al* (2002), for the HERS Research Group, "Cardiovascular disease outcomes during 6.8 years of hormone therapy," Heart and Estrogen/progestin Replacement Study follow up (HERS II), *Journal of the American Medical Association*, 288, 49–57

5. Writing Group for the Women's Health Initiative Investigators (2002), "Risks and benefits of oestrogen plus progestin in healthy postmenopausal women: principal results from the Women's Health Initiative randomised controlled trial," *Journal of the American Medical Association*, 288, 321–33

6. Elliot, W.J. *American Journal of Medicine*, 1983, 75, 1024–32

7. Clarke, R. *et al* (1998), "Lowering blood homocysteine with folic acid based supplements: Meta-analysis of randomised trials," *British Medical Journal*, 316, 894–8

8. Vermulen, E.G. *et al* (2000), "Effect of homocysteine-lowering treatment with folic acid plus vitamin B6 on progression of subclinical artherosclerosis: a randomised placebo controlled trial," *The Lancet*, 355, 517–22

9. Salonen, J.T. *et al* (1998), "Donation of blood is associated with reduced risk of myocardial infarction," The Kuopio Ischaemic Heart Disease Risk Factor Study, *American Journal of Epidemiology*, 148, 445–51

10. de Valk, B. and Marx, J.J. (1999), "Iron, atherosclerosis and ischemic heart disease," *Archives of Internal Medicine*, 159, 1542–8

11. Anderson, J. *et al*, "Meta-analysis of the effects of soy protein intake on serum lipids" (1995), *New England Journal of Medicine*, 333, 5, 276–82

12. Pratt, D.E. *et al* (1979), "Source of antioxidant activity of soybeans and soy products,"

Journal of Food Science, 44, 1720-2
13. Goodman-Gruen, D. and Kritz-Silverstein, D. (2001), "Usual dietary isoflavone intake is associated with cardiovascular disease risk factors in postmenopausal women," *Journal of Nutrition*, 131, 4, 1202-6
14. *American Journal of Clinical Nutrition* (2000), 71, 103-8
15. Stephens, N.G. *et al* (1996), "Randomised controlled trial of vitamin E in patients with coronary disease," *The Lancet*, 347, 781-6
16. Pryor, A. (2000), "Vitamin E and heart disease: basic science to clinical intervention trial," *Free Radical Biology and Medicine*, 28, 141-64

Chapter 11
1. Blundell, J.E. and Hill, A.J. (1986), "Paradoxical effects of an intense sweetener (aspartame) on appetite," *The Lancet*, 1, 1092-3
2. Neilsen, F.H. (1996), "Controversial chromium: does the superstar mineral of the Mountebanks receive appropriate attention from clinicians and nutritionists?," *Nutrition Today*, 31, 226-33
3. Evans, G.W. and Pouchnik, D.J. (1993), "Composition and biological activity of chromium-pyridine carboxylate complexes," *Journal of Inorganic Biochemistry*, 49, 177-87
4. Van Gaal, L. *et al* (1984), "Biomedical and clinical aspects of coenzyme Q10," 4, 369
5. Yamamoto, I. *et al* (1974), "Anti-tumour effects of seaweed," *Japanese Journal of Experimental Medicine*, 44, 543-6
6. Iritani, N. and Nagi, S. "Effects of spinach and wakame on cholesterol turnover in the rat," *Atherosclerosis*, 15, 87-92
7. Olivieri, O. *et al* (1995), "Low selenium status in the elderly influences thyroid hormones," *Clinical Science*, 89, 637-42

Chapter 13
1. Suzuki, T. and Yamamoto, P. (1982), "Organic mercury levels in human hair with and without storage for eleven years," *Bull Environ Contam Toxicol*, 28. 186-8
2. James, V. (1999), "Using hair to screen for breast cancer," Nature, 398, 6722, 33-4
3. Dickman, M.D. and Leung, K.M. (1998), "Mercury and organochlorine exposure from fish consumption in Hong Kong," *Chemosphere*, 37, 5, 991-1015
4. Miekeley, N. (2001), "Elemental anomalies in hair as indicators of endocrinologic pathologies and deficiencies in calcium and bone metabolism," *Journal of Trace Elem Med Biol*, 15, 1, 46-55

Index

About the Author

Dr. Marilyn Glenville, Ph.D., is a Fellow of the Royal Society of Medicine, a registered nutritionist and a psychologist who obtained her doctorate from Cambridge University.

For over 25 years, Dr. Glenville has studied and practiced nutritional therapy both in the U.K. and in the U.S., specializing in the natural approach to female hormone problems. She has had several papers published in scientific journals, frequently advises health professionals and often lectures at academic conferences. She is a popular international speaker and author of a number of best-selling books, including *Natural Alternatives to Dieting, Eat Your Way through the Menopause, Natural Solutions to Infertility* and *The Nutritional Health Handbook for Women.*

Dr. Glenville was officially appointed by the U.K.'s Foods Standards Agency as an observer on the Expert Group on Vitamins and Minerals set up by the British government to look into the safety of vitamins and minerals. She is also a steering group member of the Forum on Food and Health at the Royal Society of Medicine and a member of the Nutrition Society. She runs her own clinics in London and Tunbridge Wells, Kent.

Other Ulysses Press Mind/Body Titles

ANXIETY & DEPRESSION: A NATURAL APPROACH
2nd edition, Shirley Trickett, $10.95

A step-by-step organic solution for sufferers that puts the reader—not the drugs—in control.

ASHTANGA YOGA FOR WOMEN: INVIGORATING MIND, BODY AND SPIRIT WITH POWER YOGA
Sally Griffyn and Michaela Clarke, $17.95

Featuring 240 photographs, this is the first power yoga book designed expressly for women. Approachable and easy to use, it includes detailed, step-by-step instruction on individual as well as entire sequences.

FIBROMYALGIA: A NATURAL APPROACH
Christine Craggs Hinton, $14.95

Offers a complete self-care program for reversing the painful, debilitating symptoms of fibromyalgia—a chronic but little-understood condition affecting muscle, tendons and joints.

50 + YOGA: TIPS AND TECHNIQUES FOR A SAFE AND HEALTHY PRACTICE
Richard Rosen, $12.95

Focusing on the needs of the beginning student 50 years and older, this book details the basic principles of yoga and teaches the yoga poses through the use of step-by-step photos, clearly written instructions and helpful hints from the author.

HOW MEDITATION HEALS: A SCIENTIFIC EXPLANATION
Eric Harrison, $12.95

In straightforward, practical terms, *How Meditation Heals* reveals how and why meditation improves the natural functioning of the human body.

KNOW YOUR BODY: THE ATLAS OF ANATOMY
2nd edition, Introduction by Emmet B. Keeffe, M.D., $14.95

Provides a comprehensive, full-color guide to the human body.

101 SIMPLE WAYS TO MAKE YOUR HOME & FAMILY SAFE IN A TOXIC WORLD
Beth Ann Petro Roybal, $11.95

Sheds light on common toxins found around the house and offers parents straightforward ways to protect themselves and their children.

PILATES WORKBOOK: ILLUSTRATED STEP-BY-STEP GUIDE
TO MATWORK TECHNIQUES
Michael King, $12.95

Illustrates the core matwork movements exactly as Joseph Pilates intended them to be performed; readers learn each movement by simply following the photographic sequences and explanatory captions.

SENSES WIDE OPEN: THE ART & PRACTICE OF LIVING IN YOUR BODY
Johanna Putnoi, $14.95

Through simple, accessible exercises, this book shows how to be at ease with yourself and experience genuine pleasure in your physical connection to others and the world.

THE 7 HEALING CHAKRAS: UNLOCKING YOUR BODY'S ENERGY CENTERS
Dr. Brenda Davies, $14.95

Explores the essence of chakras—vortices of energy that connect the physical body with the spiritual.

TEACH YOURSELF TO MEDITATE IN 10 SIMPLE LESSONS: DISCOVER
RELAXATION AND CLARITY OF MIND IN JUST MINUTES A DAY
Eric Harrison, $12.95

Guides the reader through ten easy-to-follow core meditations. Also included are practical and enjoyable "spot meditations" that require only a few minutes a day and can be incorporated into the busiest of schedules.

YOGA THERAPIES: 45 SEQUENCES TO RELIEVE STRESS, DEPRESSION,
REPETITIVE STRAIN, SPORTS INJURIES AND MORE
Jessie Chapman   Photographs by Dhyan, $14.95

Featuring an inspiring artistic presentation, this book is filled with beautifully photographed sequences that relieve stress, release anger, relax back muscles and reverse repetitive strain injuries.

To order these books call 800-377-2542 or 510-601-8301, fax 510-601-8307, e-mail ulysses@ulyssespress.com, or write to Ulysses Press, P.O. Box 3440, Berkeley, CA 94703. All retail orders are shipped free of charge. California residents must include sales tax. Allow two to three weeks for delivery.

Staying in Touch

If you have any health problems and are interested in finding a more natural approach to treating them, or would like to find out what supplements and tests are available to you, please feel free to contact my clinic for information on how you can help yourself.

Workshops
I am invited to give many workshops and talks around the world. Please call or check my website if you would like to find out whether I will be speaking at a location near you, and you will also be sent an information pack. If you would like to organize a talk or workshop in your area, please call or email for details.

Tests and Products
If you are having problems obtaining or would like more information about any of the products or tests mentioned in this book, please contact www.naturalhealthpractice.com. Here you will find everything I recommend in the book and much more.

Consultations
If you would like help with any personal health problems, private consultations are available at my London or Tunbridge Wells clinics. Postal consultations are also available. For appointments and inquiries contact:

Dr. Glenville, 14 St. John's Road, Tunbridge Wells, Kent, TN4 9NP UK
Tel: 0870 5329244 / Fax: 0870 5329255
Int Tel: 011 44 1892 505 905 / Int Fax: 011 44 1892 515 914
Website: www.marilynglenville.com
Email: health@marilynglenville.com